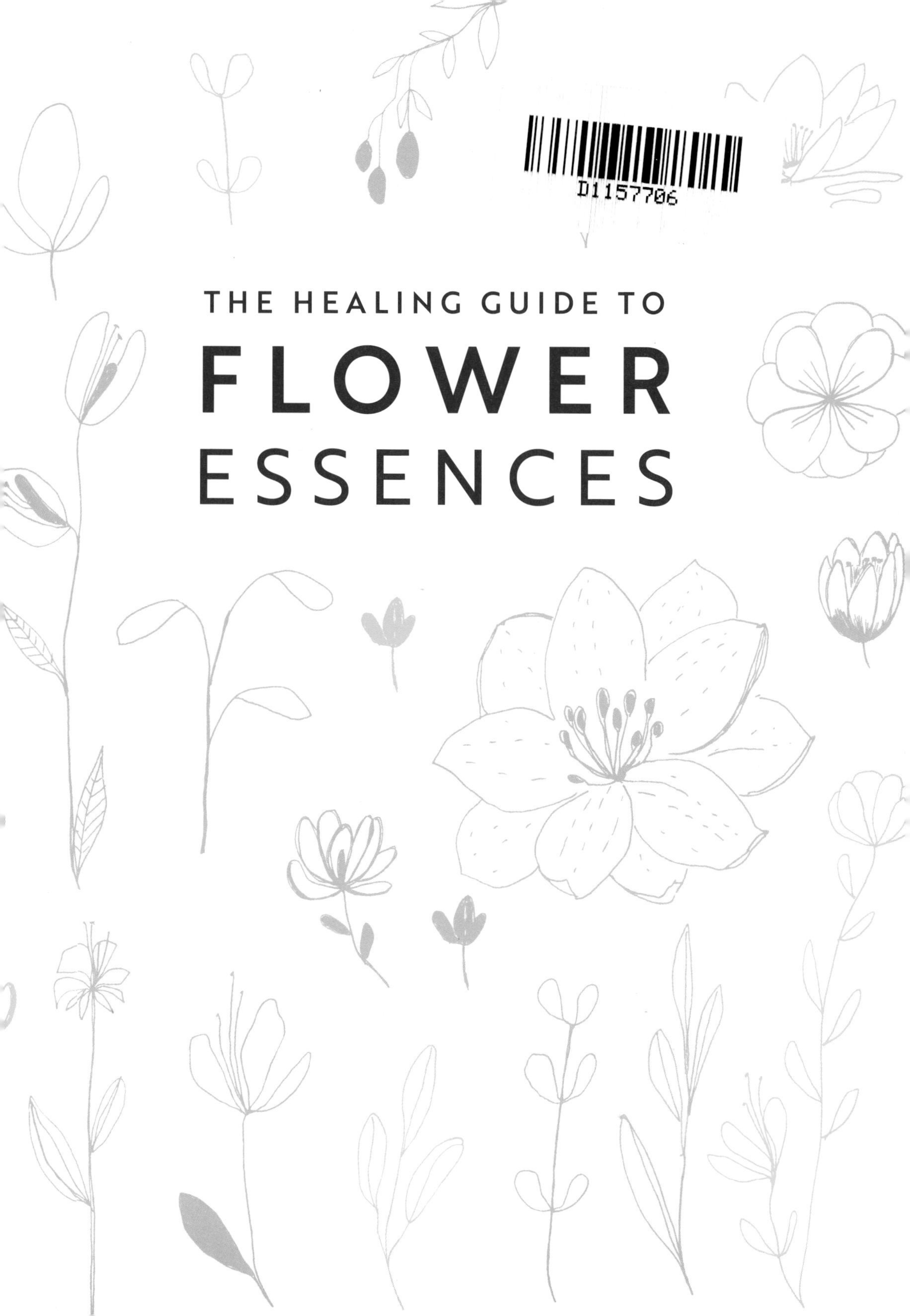

THE HEALING GUIDE TO FLOWER ESSENCES

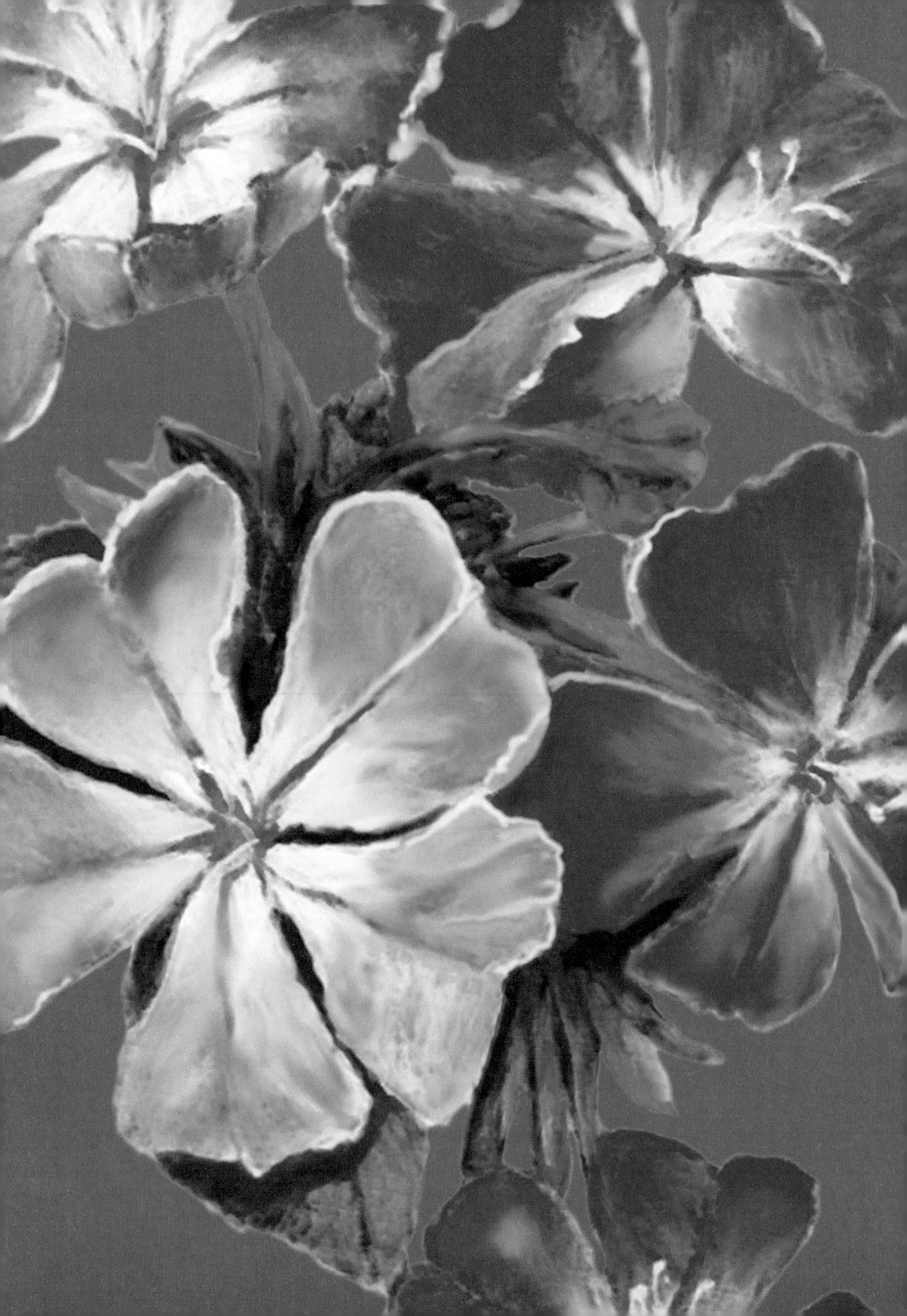

THE HEALING GUIDE TO FLOWER ESSENCES

How to Use Gaia's Magick and Medicine for Wellness, Transformation, and Emotional Balance

ALENA HENNESSY

WITH ART BY

Jane Hennessy

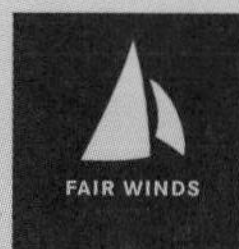

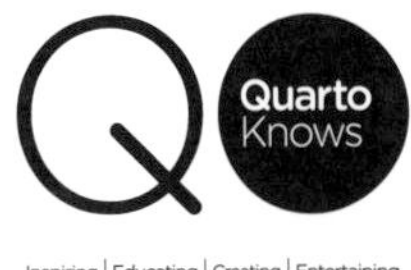

Brimming with creative inspiration, how-to projects, and useful information to enrich your everyday life, Quarto Knows is a favorite destination for those pursuing their interests and passions. Visit our site and dig deeper with our books into your area of interest: Quarto Creates, Quarto Cooks, Quarto Homes, Quarto Lives, Quarto Drives, Quarto Explores, Quarto Gifts, or Quarto Kids.

First Published in 2020 by Fair Winds Press, an imprint of The Quarto Group,
100 Cummings Center, Suite 265-D, Beverly, MA 01915, USA.
T (978) 282-9590 F (978) 283-2742 QuartoKnows.com

Fair Winds Press titles are also available at discount for retail, wholesale, promotional, and bulk purchase. For details, contact the Special Sales Manager by email at specialsales@quarto.com or by mail at The Quarto Group, Attn: Special Sales Manager, 100 Cummings Center, Suite 265-D, Beverly, MA 01915, USA.

24 23 22 21 20   1 2 3 4 5

ISBN: 978-1-59233-938-9

Digital edition published in 2020
eISBN: 978-1-63159-853-1

Library of Congress Cataloging-in-Publication Data is available.

Design & Layout: Tanya Jacobson, jcbsn.co
Illustration: all flowers, Jane Hennessy; all line art and backgrounds, Alena Hennessy

Printed in Malaysia

DISCLAIMER

Flower essences are universally known to be safe to ingest; however, please double-check to make sure the flower you choose for your essence is indeed the right one (other, similar-looking flowers can be poisonous). Poisonous plants can be used for flower essences, yet unlike herbal remedies or essential oils, extremely tiny amounts of plant matter are in the formula. Essentially, do your research to make sure that the exact species you've chosen is safe to touch and work with, and also be careful to make sure it has not been sprayed with pesticides or the like. If you are unsure, err on the side of caution and buy a ready-made flower essence from an established maker.

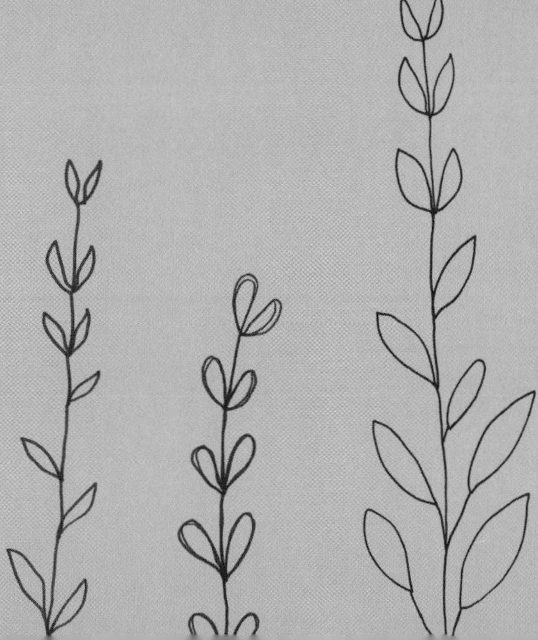

CONTENTS

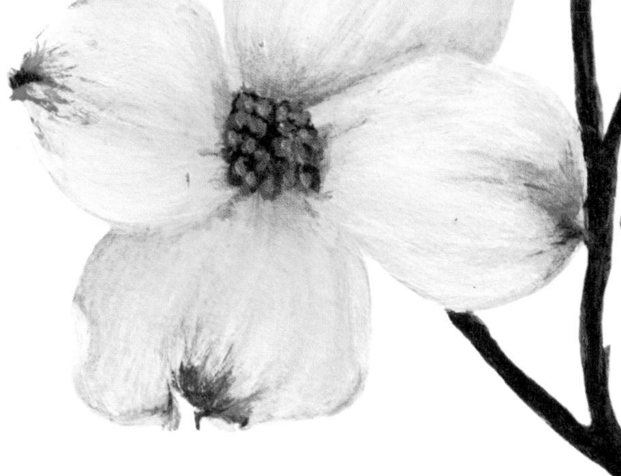

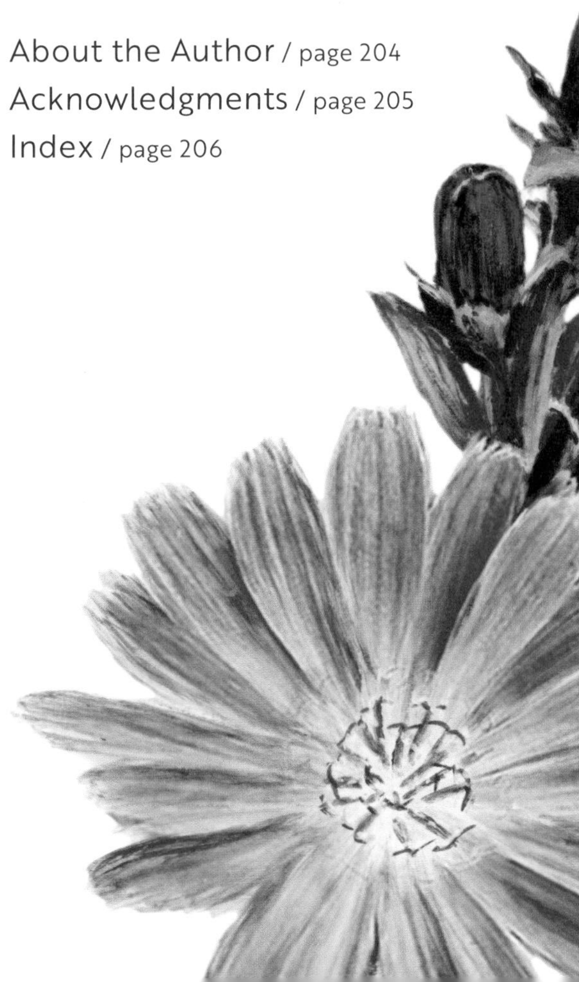

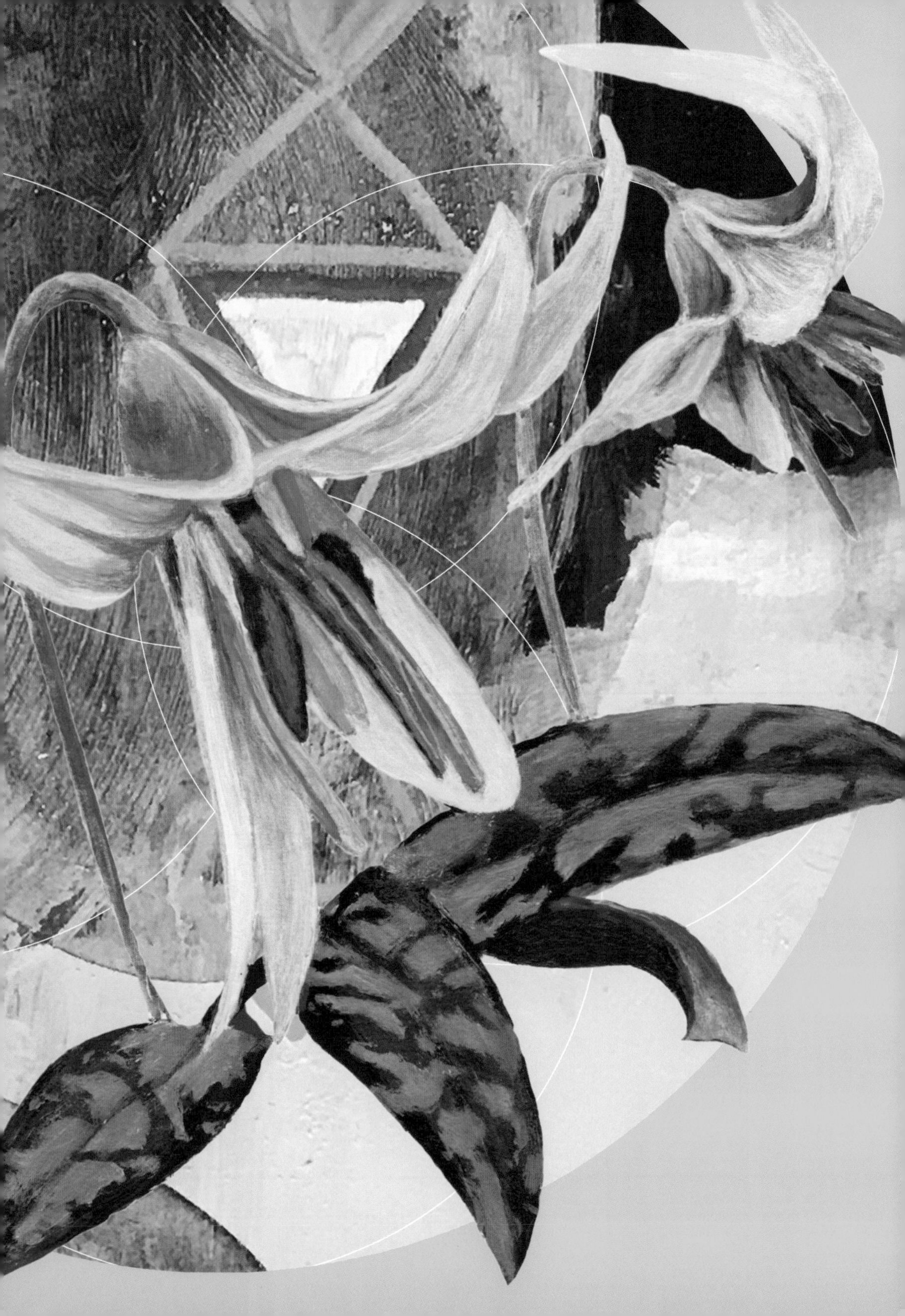

1 What Flower Essences Actually Are

Flower essences are infusions of the energetic qualities of flowers. They address the nature and wellness of one's soul and emotions, as well as the connection to one's whole being.

Flower essences are made from freshly picked flowers held in spring or distilled water by the sun or light of the moon. After their vibrational medicine is infused into the water, they are diluted further, potentized, and preserved in glass jars and dropper bottles for ingestion.

Flower remedies are a gentle or subtle medicine. That means they work on deeper layers of the emotional body and our subconscious for integration into the soul's well-being. The essences are a homeopathic medicine, meaning they work with the main imprinting of pain or trauma, where the imbalance is held within the body. For example, if you are working with low self-esteem, the energetic imprint of the essence works to build confidence and self-worth, and insecure emotions are lowered. Subtle shifts in our energy can cause ripples in our lives for a beautiful and gentle transformational process. When healing takes place in a gentle energy field, as the flowers so sweetly provide, it can be brought into union gracefully with the mind-body-spirit connection and ourselves. The effects of the essence sometimes can be felt right away; other times, subtle shifts unfold day by day until there is a change.

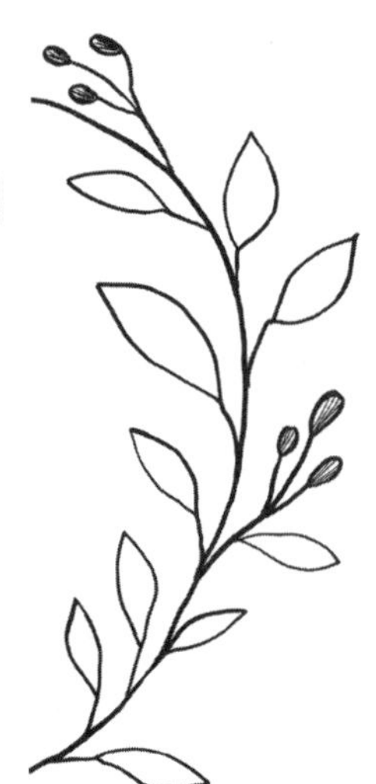

Flower Essences, Essential Oils, and Herbal Tinctures
Flower essences are not to be confused with essential oils or herbal tinctures. Essential oils are chemical compounds from a plant extracted in a distillation process. They're often used for aromatherapy because of their potent smell. An herbal tincture is a concentrated medicinal form of a plant that is made by soaking it in alcohol for an extended period of time. Tinctures are used to help heal and balance physical symptoms in the body.

A Little History

Utilizing flowers for their subtle yet transformative powers of healing dates back almost 3,000 years and has occurred in many cultures throughout the world. The ancient Egyptians were known to collect the dew from flowers and use its energetic properties to treat intense emotional states. For centuries, the Chinese have been known to embrace the energetic vibrations of flowers as beneficial for one's well-being. The Balinese have a long history of placing flowers in bathwater and taking a long soak for beauty and rejuvenation.

Hildegard von Bingen (1098–1179), a mystic, writer, composer, and Benedictine abbess from Germany, was a highly in-tune visionary who later came to be known as Saint Hildegard. She wrote texts about the medicinal, theological, and elemental healing properties of botany and the natural world. She, along with her fellow nuns, would place muslin cloths over flowers to soak up dew. Hildegard had an innate understanding of the doctrine of signatures, the idea that parts of nature, including flowers, have direct counterparts in the human body and can assist in providing restoration and relief. The nuns would collect the muslin in the morning and use it to wrap ill patients as necessary.

The Swiss physician, alchemist, prophet, and botanist Paracelsus (1493–1541) was a radical medical practitioner because of his views on health and nature. He looked to nature as a true healer instead of the accepted paradigm, which was less holistic. Paracelsus understood the doctrine of signatures philosophy as well; he collected dew from the flowers to treat emotional imbalance, for instance. Paracelsus appreciated the flowers' innate ability to provide health to the human body.

Centuries later, the true father of flower essences was Dr. Edward Bach (1886–1936). Bach was a dedicated physician from London who understood that traditional medicine, or allopathic practices, has its limitations in providing well-being. Dr. Bach became drawn to a homeopathic approach, one in which he embraced the healing power of flowers. He began to collect wildflowers with which to treat patients and noticed positive results. He continued to study and reflect upon the gifts of each of these flowers, as related to treating human beings. To quote Dr. Bach about the magnificent power of flower essence healing:

> “*. . . To raise our vibrations and open up our channels for the reception of our spiritual self, to flood our natures with the particular virtues and to wash out from us the faults which were causing them. They are able, like beautiful music or any gloriously uplifting thing which gives us inspiration, to raise our very natures and bring us nearer to ourselves and by that very act to bring us peace and relieve our suffering. They cure not by attacking disease but by flooding our bodies with beautiful vibrations of our higher nature in the presence of which disease melts as snow in the sunshine.*

In the 1930s, he left his successful medical practice and focused solely on working with flowers and their doctrine of signatures for treating patients. He innately understood that his patients' physical ailments were related to unintegrated charges from emotional and mental states. To make flower essences, Dr. Bach would place a flower in a glass bowl with water and let it soak for several hours. The water would receive the energetic imprint of that flower's healing capacity. We still use this method today.

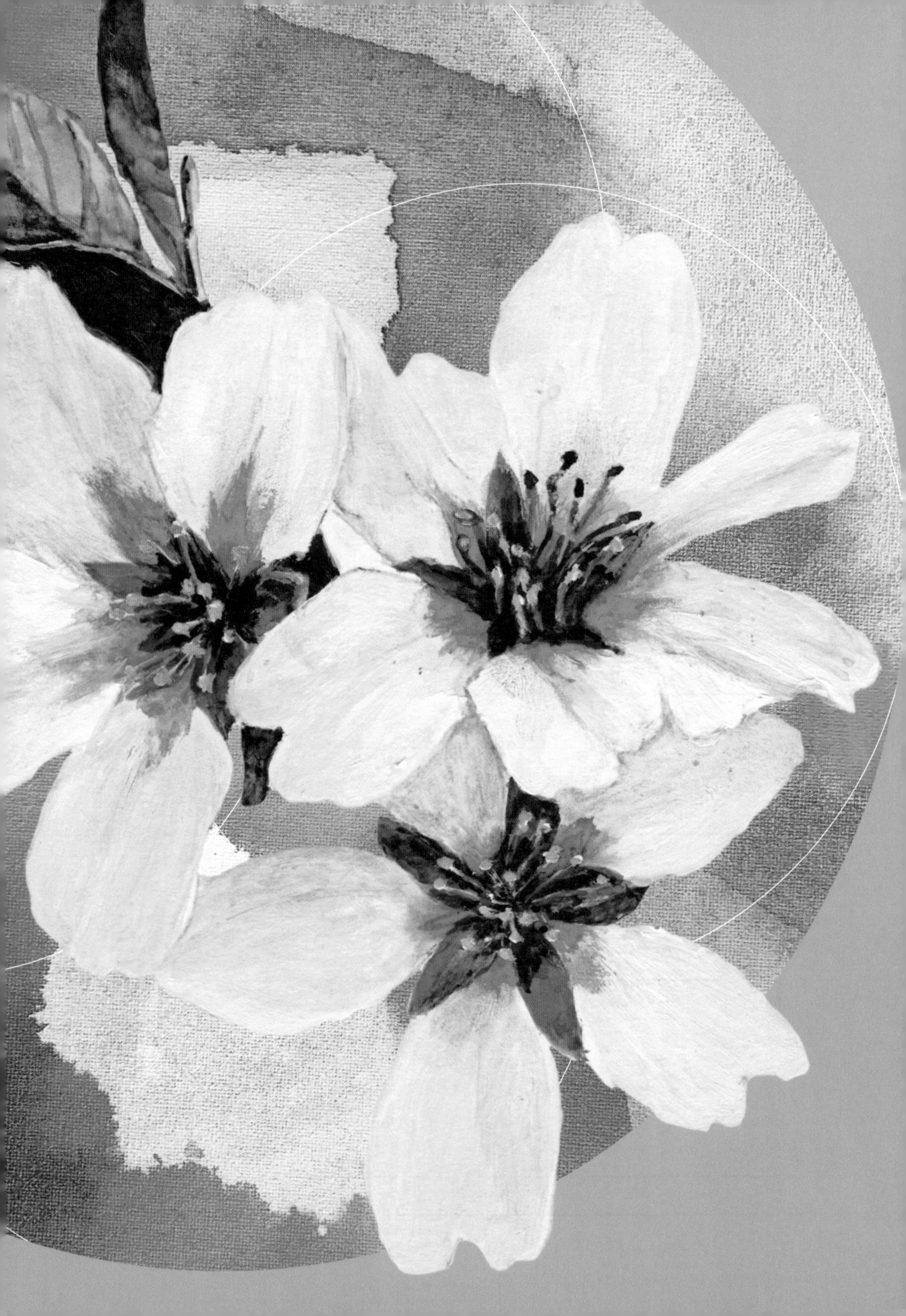

2 Dr. Bach's 38 Essential Remedies

Dr. Bach created a foundation of essential remedies for flower essences, each representing healing powers of vibration for certain characters or negative emotional states. Here are some of the plants he worked with and the negative characteristics they help address:

- **Agrimony:** suffering behind a happy demeanor
- **Aspen:** fear of the unknown
- **Beech:** irritability and lack of compassion
- **Centaury:** lack of boundaries
- **Cerato:** doubting easily
- **Cherry Plum:** fear of losing control
- **Chestnut Bud:** repetition of harmful patterns
- **Chicory:** high expectations in love
- **Clematis:** constant thoughts of the future
- **Crab Apple:** self-loathing
- **Elm:** easily overwhelmed nature
- **Gentian:** feeling discouraged
- **Gorse:** deep despair
- **Heather:** excessive self-interest
- **Holly:** jealousy and aggressive feelings toward others
- **Honeysuckle:** overly nostalgic sentiments
- **Hornbeam:** feelings of exhaustion about tasks
- **Impatiens:** lack of patience
- **Larch:** lack of self-esteem
- **Mimulus:** fear of things known
- **Mustard:** deep depression
- **Oak:** refusal to rest and self-care
- **Olive:** feeling of exhaustion after efforts made
- **Pine:** blaming oneself
- **Red Chestnut:** excessive worry about loved ones
- **Rock Rose:** intense fear and shock
- **Rock Water:** being too hard on oneself
- **Scleranthus:** indecisiveness
- **Star of Bethlehem:** crisis
- **Sweet Chestnut:** intense mental anguish
- **Vervain:** being overly persuasive with one's point of view
- **Vine:** being domineering and intolerant of others
- **Walnut:** in need of protection from outside influences
- **Water Violet:** tendency to isolate
- **White Chestnut:** anxiety and repetitive thinking
- **Wild Oat:** feeling unsure about what path to take
- **Wild Rose:** feeling resigned or apathetic
- **Willow:** bitterness and resentment

How to Make Your Own Flower Essences

Making your own flower essences is a wonderful practice that connects you further to the magical and soothing energy of flower essences. When making your own remedies, you become your own practitioner and alchemist. The transformation and healing begin as soon as you sit and begin to prepare the flower remedy.

Note: Brandy is the usual preservative, but try apple cider vinegar if you are sensitive to alcohol.

Materials Needed:

- Glass bowl
- Spring or distilled water
- Scissors and/or tweezers
- Mesh strainer (or coffee filter/cheesecloth)
- Glass jar with lid such as a mason jar
- Brandy, organic alcohol, distilled white vinegar, vegetable glycerin, or apple cider vinegar for preserving
- Labels
- Small glass dropper bottle

It's best to choose a day on which there will be ample sunshine, so heading out in the morning is best. Go to a field or forest where wildflowers grow, a park, or your own garden. Choose a flower that is growing and speaking to you right now, and choose just one species. *Before choosing flowers for your remedy, always ask the flowers' permission and if they desire to be picked.* You may also wish to ask them for any messages they have about their healing properties and purpose. You will be delightfully surprised by what you receive. This is a beloved and precious moment, and you are making a heart connection with the plant.

Once you have decided which flowers to work with, set up your glass bowl next to the plant and fill it with spring water. Cut or tweeze the flowers at the base. Place them in an even row, covering the surface of the water with flowers faceup. Do not cover up the bowl. Be aware throughout this process. Meditate and share your intentions with the healing powers of these flowers. You are the medicine maker! Offer gratitude for the flowers and for this process.

Allow the flowers to sit in the bowl with the spring water for 3 to 4 hours in sunlight. Then carefully remove the flowers and strain the water into a clear glass jar with a 50:50 ratio of flower water and preservative of your choice. This is the *mother essence* of one particular flower. Label the jar with the flower, the date, and any intentions or messages that came through.

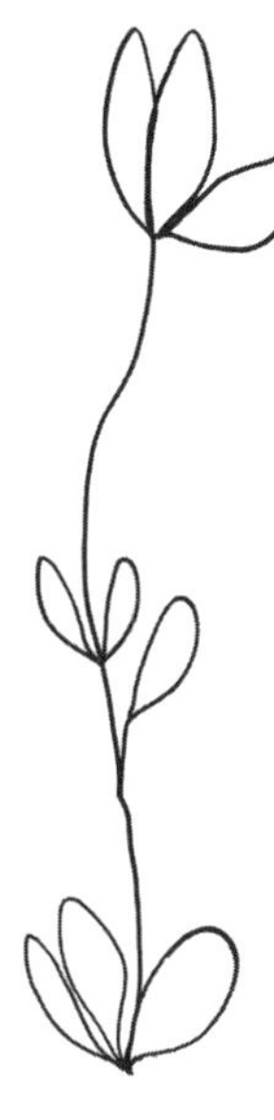

Disclaimer
Please double-check to make sure the flower you are choosing for your essence is indeed the right one (other, similar-looking flowers can be poisonous). Do your research to make sure that the exact species you've chosen is safe to touch and work with, and also be careful to make sure it has not been sprayed with pesticides or the like. If you are unsure, err on the side of caution and buy a ready-made flower essence from an established maker.

To make your stock bottle (which is what you can buy in stores and online), add 4 to 7 drops of the mother essence to a small glass amber dropper bottle filled with a 50:50 ratio of spring water to the preservative of your choice. The reason so few drops are used is similar to the philosophy of homeopathy. When you dilute the essence, you are making the essence smaller and therefore more potent for the deeper energetic layers you wish to address. After making your stock bottle, you may tap or shake it to activate its energetic properties.

If you wish, you can begin to build a variety of stock bottles from your mother essences to keep on hand. Then create specific dosage bottles that each contain 1 to 5 essences you wish to take, depending on what you need at a given time. Simply put 2 drops from each stock bottle essence in that dosage bottle, then fill the bottle with ¼ to ½ ounce of brandy to preserve it. (Again, if you do not want to use alcohol as a preservative, you may use apple cider vinegar or vegetable glycerin.) If you are new to flower essences, start working with one essence at time and then build up from there.

How to Take Flower Essences

You can take flower essences in a variety of ways. Typically, you take them orally from the stock bottles you buy online or in health food stores. The standard dosage is up to 4 drops in your mouth up to 4 times a day. However, you can also sip water with your flower essence drops in it (4 drops per large glass of water). Put the drops of essence in a glass of water and sip throughout the day. You also may use flower essences in spritzers, creams, lotions, baths, and so forth.

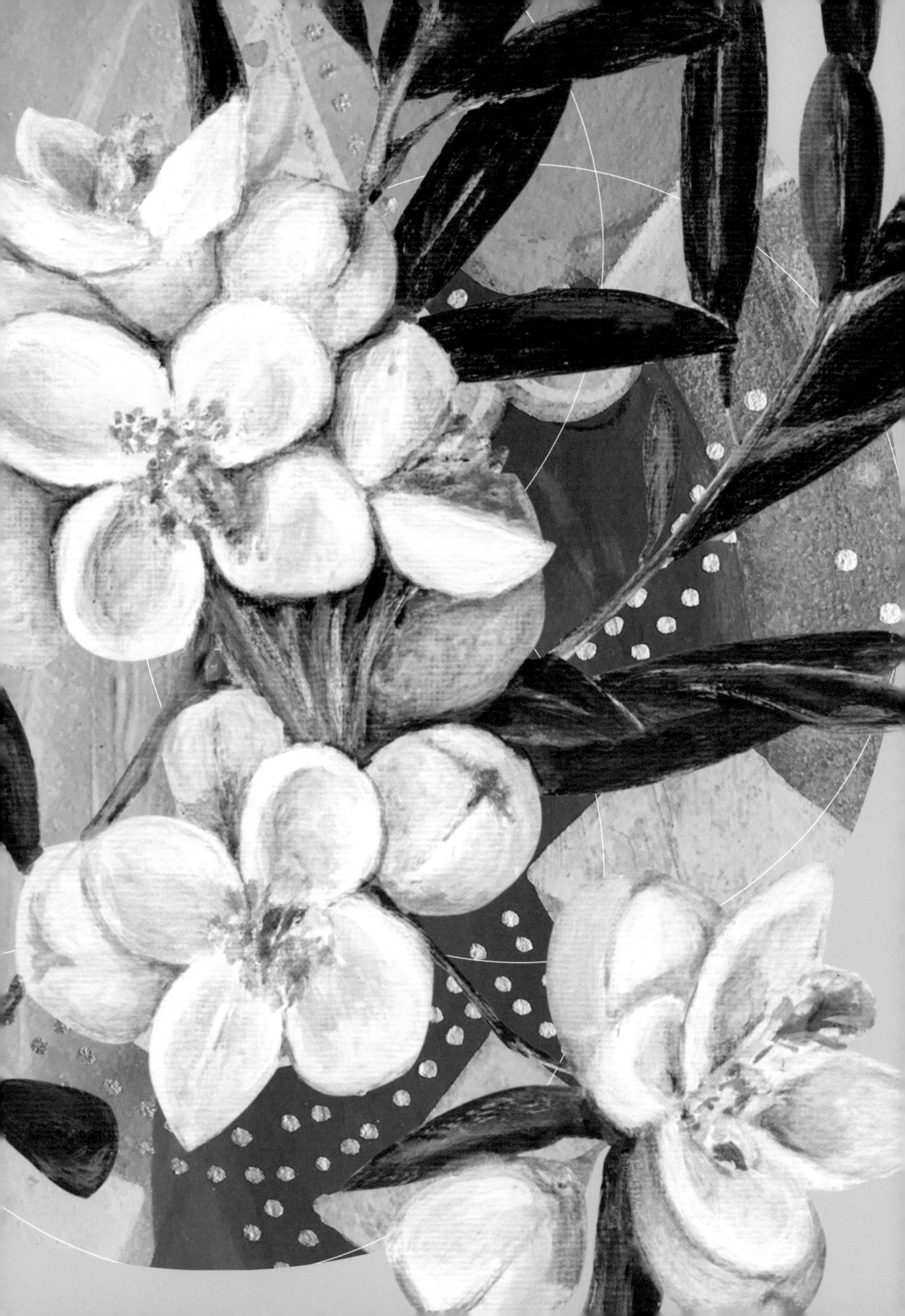

3 Flower Essences for Anxiety

If you want to conquer the anxiety of life, live in the moment, live in the breath.

— Amit Ray

Some say we live in an age of anxiety. We have become a society that has succumbed to information overload. Thanks to the ever-expanding influence of social media and 24/7 news outlets, our lives are full of constant interactions, distractions, and anxiety. Anxiety activates the nervous system within the body. With the bombardment of smartphones, laptops, and tablets, it is easy to see why so many of us feel chronically anxious and overwhelmed. There is always another news story to pay attention to, email to answer, or message that needs a response. And what happens when we have situations or emotions we don't know how to manage? All too often we scroll through the latest social media postings to mindlessly distract ourselves.

So what are some helpful antidotes to calm our inner world? Learning to meditate, spending time in nature, exercising, reducing or eliminating caffeine and other stimulants, and spending less time on our phones can all help alleviate anxious states. The other wonderful news is that many flower essences can assist us in living a more centered, peaceful, anxiety-free life. Call upon the flower essences listed below to allow the mind and body to realign with the natural rhythm of life. From there may you breathe into a fuller relaxation of existence.

Aloe Vera

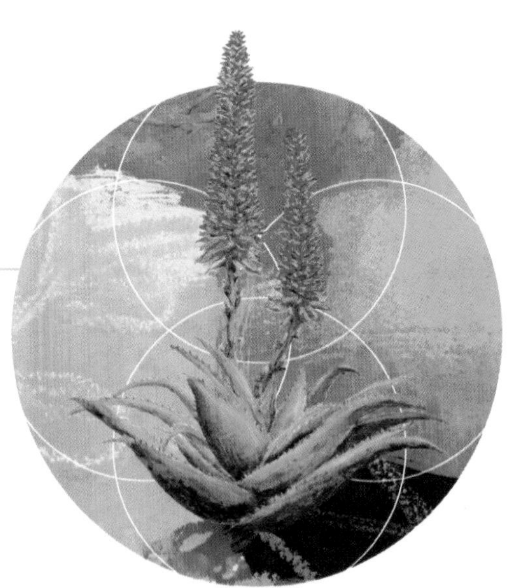

ALOE VERA FLOWER ESSENCE WILL ASSIST YOU WITH:

- Balancing overly ambitious patterns
- Soothing a fiery nature
- Rejuvenating the spirit

Invocation

Dip your feet into some cool water and take this flower essence to calm an overdriven nature. The Aloe Vera flower essence will help with burnout and restore balance from overwork. Allow it to guide you in harmonizing the time allotted for work, rest, and play.

Aloe Vera, an evergreen perennial, grows wild in tropical climates all over the world. This plant has many medicinal uses both internally and topically. This potent flower essence is helpful to those who are experiencing mental and physical exhaustion from burning the candle at both ends. People who are fiery in nature and have fallen into a pattern of anxious workaholism would benefit from taking Aloe Vera. Their inner drive has taken over, and they have forgotten their other physical, spiritual, and emotional needs. This obsessive determination overrides the ability to experience life from the heart and thus deprives the body-mind-spirit connection of feeling in harmony with the inherent nature and balance of things. Aloe Vera flower essence restores that balance, enabling the life force to return to states of vitality and centeredness. Restoration and rejuvenation are some more gifts that Aloe Vera brings, helping you to remember to work from a place of positivity that is sourced from the heart. Willpower then comes into harmony with the flow of life, bringing about more centered productivity and a sense of well-being.

Chamomile

CHAMOMILE FLOWER ESSENCE WILL ASSIST YOU WITH:

- Finding serenity
- Balancing moody emotions
- Embodying a sunny outlook

Invocation

On a sunny day, go walk out in nature and take Chamomile flower essence to restore a positive disposition. This flower essence is perfect to take when you have been feeling extra moody or irritable.

Chamomile, belonging to the Asteraceae or daisy family, is an annual wild edible that is native to parts of Europe, India, and western Asia. It is a common herbal remedy for relaxation before bedtime and has a long, rich history of medicinal properties. A person who would benefit from taking Chamomile flower essence is one who is easily irritable, anxious, and unable to let go of emotional imbalance or bad moods. This flower essence is also good for those who often experience mood swings and constant fluctuation in their emotional body. Those who often hold emotional tension in their stomachs would also benefit from taking this essence. It can even be used with children who experience a wide range of moods throughout the day. Chamomile flower essence can help treat insomnia because a soul suffering from emotional tension can have trouble becoming calm at night. This flower essence can bring about a more equanimous and serene state, giving an individual deeper peace and stability within.

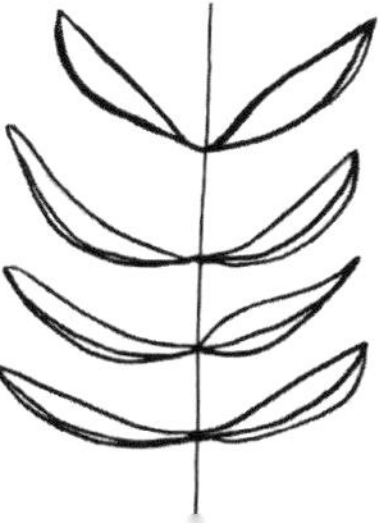

Cherry Plum

CHERRY PLUM FLOWER ESSENCE WILL ASSIST YOU WITH:

- Finding balance and calm during intense stress
- Feeling trustful again
- Surrendering to a Higher Power

Invocation

Take this flower essence when everything feels like it's falling apart. Remember that you are more than enough and that you are going to be okay. Light candles, put on some relaxing music, and take Cherry Plum flower essence. Allow equanimity to enter your state of being.

Cherry Plum, native to southeast Europe and western Asia, is a large shrub or tall, spiny tree with deciduous leaves. This flower essence is appropriate for anyone experiencing anxiety, fear, or destructive emotional patterns. Cherry Plum also could help those going through intense stress and psychological or emotional breakdowns. This flower essence is suitable for people afraid of losing control and spiraling in a downward direction. Cherry Plum assists in the soul's ability to trust again and in feeling higher guidance and states of balance. The energy of Cherry Plum is that of surrender so that it can stabilize and ground the whole person. Cherry Plum bestows the gifts of courage, strength, and deeper states of trust.

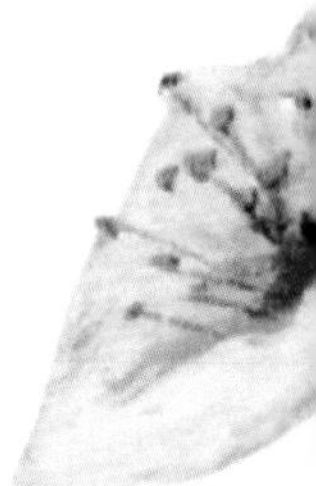

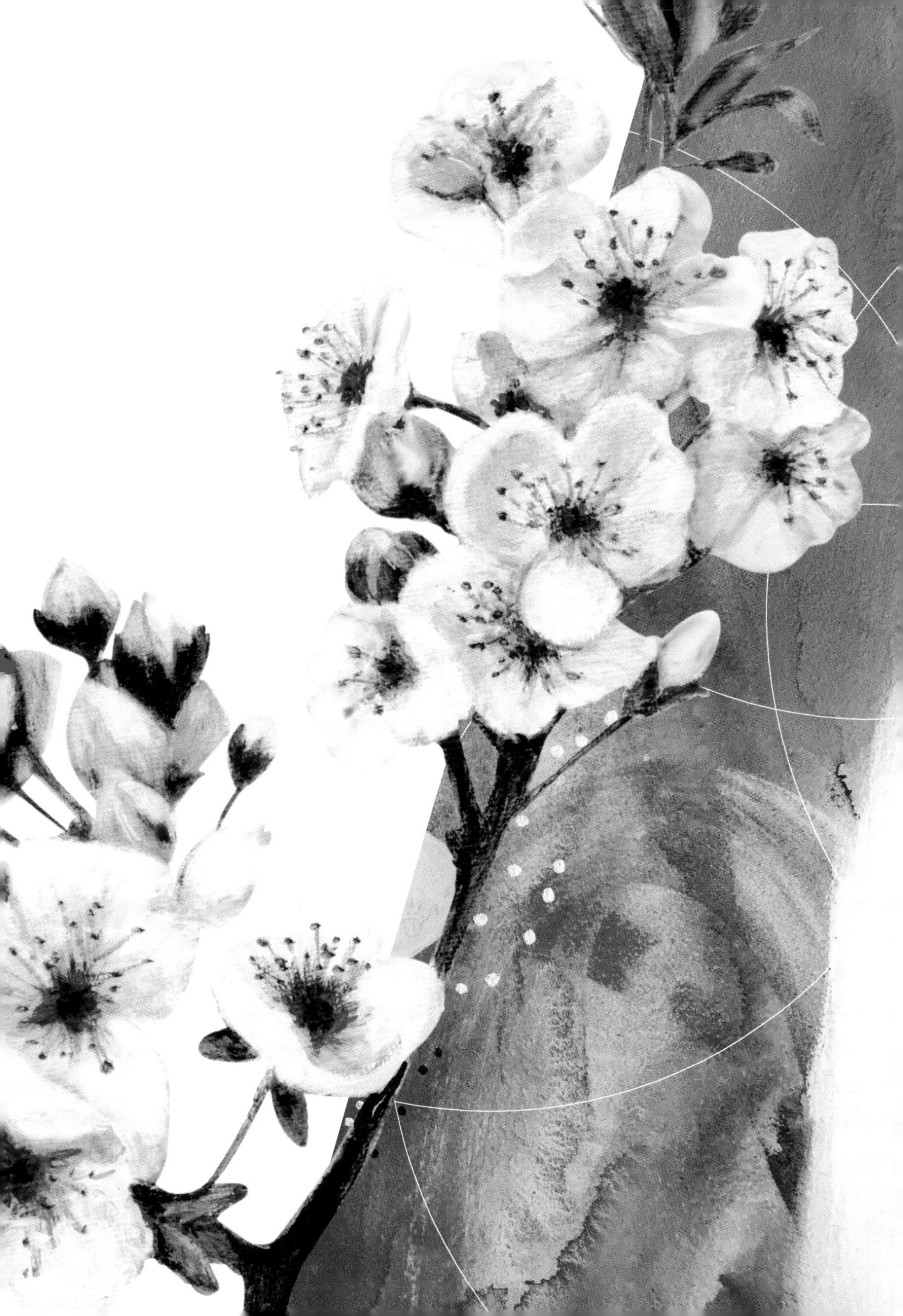

Lavender

LAVENDER FLOWER ESSENCE WILL ASSIST YOU WITH:

- Soothing nervousness
- Regulating feelings of oversensitivity
- Balancing psychic energy with physical needs of the body

Invocation

Before sitting down to meditate, take this flower essence to bring equanimity to the mind and body. Lavender flower essence is appropriate for those who are highly sensitive and intuitive or who can experience highly active mental states.

Lavender, a sweet-smelling plant known for its relaxing qualities, is native to the Mediterranean. It has evergreen leaves and soft, aromatic purple buds and prefers drier climates and soil. As a flower essence, Lavender assists those who are feeling anxious and overstimulated. It is especially helpful when nervous states begin to tax the physical body. This essence is a healer for empaths, or those who take on energetic qualities of people and the world around them. Lavender also helps those who feel overly sensitive or high-strung, experience insomnia, or often have shoulder or neck pain. This essence brings about feelings of serenity and balance for the psychic energies and physical well-being of the body.

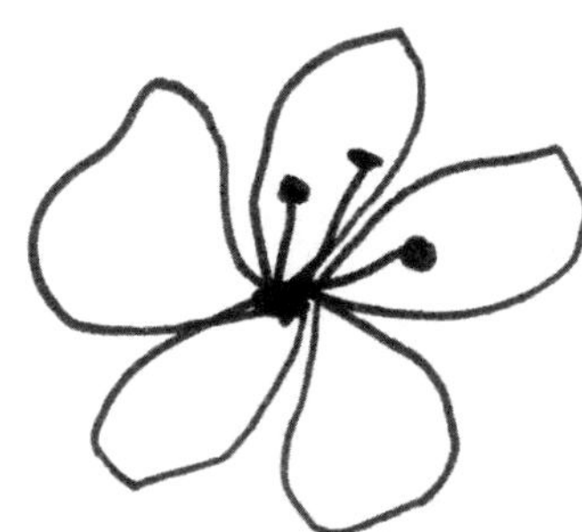

Mimulus

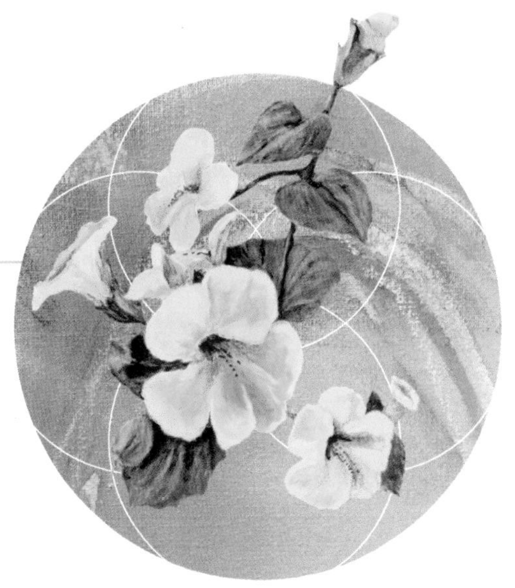

MIMULUS FLOWER ESSENCE WILL ASSIST YOU WITH:

- Overcoming fear and anxiety
- Building security within
- Tapping into courage and strength

Invocation

Write down some intentions for overcoming daily fears and anxieties when taking this flower essence. Mimulus helps sensitive souls feel brave when facing daily tasks. Know that you can feel your inner purpose with confidence now.

Mimulus, a plant that takes many forms and has yellow, tubular flowers, is native throughout parts of western North America. This flower essence assists in everyday facing of fears and anxiety. Mimulus inspires us to feel braver and more secure when facing life's challenges. Those who are especially sensitive and live with various daily fears would benefit from taking Mimulus. This brightly colored bloom helps individuals feel the light of courage within, along with a higher purpose for living. Confidence, strength, and happiness are all gifts of Mimulus. Taking this healing essence can liberate and encourage one to take risks to receive more reward in life.

Olive

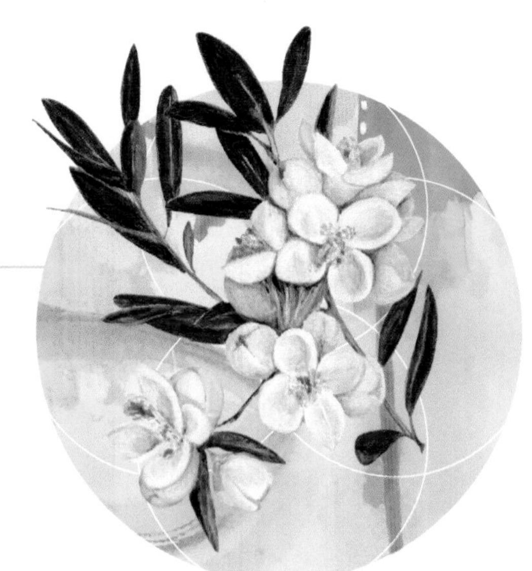

OLIVE FLOWER ESSENCE WILL ASSIST YOU WITH:

- Opening up to high states of consciousness
- Restoring the body from physical exhaustion
- Revitalizing the soul with rest

Invocation

Take this flower essence when you are overwhelmed and physically depleted. Take the Olive flower essence while partaking in a hot bath with Epsom salts and your favorite essential oils. Allow this essence to restore all your energetic and emotional bodies. Come home to your higher self.

Belonging to the family Oleaceae, Olive comes from a species of small trees found in southern Asia, China, the Arabian Peninsula, and throughout the Mediterranean Basin. Olive as a flower essence is helpful in deeply restoring the body and consciousness back into balance. It helps relieve physical stress and exhaustion while opening up states of spiritual consciousness. Olive can be understood as a gateway essence to deeper metaphysical experiences and knowledge. This flower essence assists in a soul's understanding that healing and restoration do not happen just in the body but also in one's state of mind and awareness. Olive brings in the gifts of knowing that the self is more than just a body, and one can connect to more expansive states of consciousness. From there a soul can deeply revitalize and renew.

Passionflower

PASSIONFLOWER FLOWER ESSENCE WILL ASSIST YOU WITH:

- Easing anxiety
- Inspiring intuition
- Filling your heart with divine love

Invocation

When the wear and tear of daily living is getting to your soul, allow this flower essence to be your balm. Sit down outside in nature or in a quiet area and place your hand over your heart. Take Passionflower essence slowly and feel the sensation of a relaxed and open being. Allow divine love to fill your heart and permeate all parts of your being. Rest deeply, knowing you are held in it.

Passionflower is a semi-evergreen vine with fragrant leaves that is native to South America. Medicinal tea made with its flower is said to alleviate stress, insomnia, and anxiety. The flower essence, however, also assists with lifting anxious and nervous states. Passionflower essence can inspire spiritual depth and insight. That is, it can open up channels within the body that connect to more powerful energy sources and bring about feelings of compassion and unconditional love. The flower has been a symbol of both Christ and Krishna, masters who ascended to bring a message of truth and eternal love within and in all. This powerful essence helps lift people into higher states of consciousness, away from the daily grind of anxious worldly living.

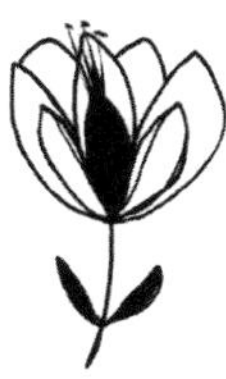

White Chestnut

WHITE CHESTNUT FLOWER ESSENCE WILL ASSIST YOU WITH:

- Quieting mental chatter
- Feeling clarity
- Balancing the energy centers

Invocation

Before going to bed, pour yourself a relaxing cup of tea (such as Passionflower or Chamomile) and take this flower essence to calm the mind. White Chestnut flower essence is for those who sometimes suffer from insomnia or busy mental chatter. Allow this essence to feed all your energy centers in a balanced way.

Native to southeast Europe, White Chestnut flower essence comes from a large deciduous tree that can grow over 100 feet (30 m) tall. This healing essence is used to calm an anxious and obsessive mind, in which mental chatter does not seem to let up. White Chestnut can help alleviate thoughts that repeat and cause excessive anxiety. That level of mental distraction can leave the physical body drained and cause insomnia and headaches. If you find yourself analyzing and worrying about your day each night as you wind down, White Chestnut may help heal some of those patterns. This essence inspires inner calm, clarity, and quiet within. Stuck energetic patterns inside the mind are redistributed throughout the body so that one can feel again through a more heart-centered way. That rational mind is brought back into balance so the intuitive mind can also be utilized. Take White Chestnut if you often find yourself facing excessive worry and repetitive thoughts.

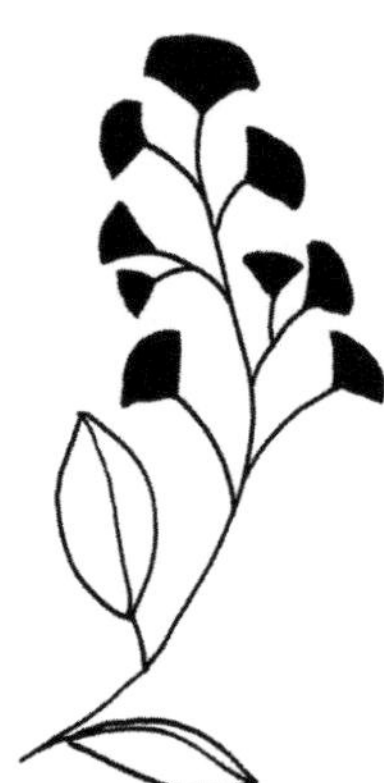

Yarrow

YARROW FLOWER ESSENCE WILL ASSIST YOU WITH:

- Protection from outside energies or toxins
- Strengthening radiance
- Building compassion and empathy

Invocation

Before preparing for travel or being surrounded by large groups of people, take this flower essence for energetic protection. The gift of Yarrow flower essence is that it also expands your warmth and radiance, allowing for inclusivity and compassion. This essence is a favorite for many practitioners because of its integrating qualities.

Yarrow, belonging to the Asteraceae family, is native to the temperate areas of Asia, North America, and Europe. The flower essence of Yarrow helps provide a field of energetic protection around a person. Yarrow is helpful in soothing stress, anxiety, and vulnerability related to the environmental toxins or negative forces coming from people or conditions. For those easily affected by others' psychic states or negativity, Yarrow is a helpful remedy that allows an individual to feel strong and sovereign despite those interactions. Take Yarrow for protection before air travel, a long drive, or a big event. This particular flower essence is good for almost everyone because it protects the soul and allows one's inner radiance to shine out naturally. Healers, empaths, teachers, counselors, and the like also will find a wonderful benefit in taking this essence. Yarrow brings about a kind healing force and stability to the energetic centers of the body, while providing room for the true self to shine out into the world.

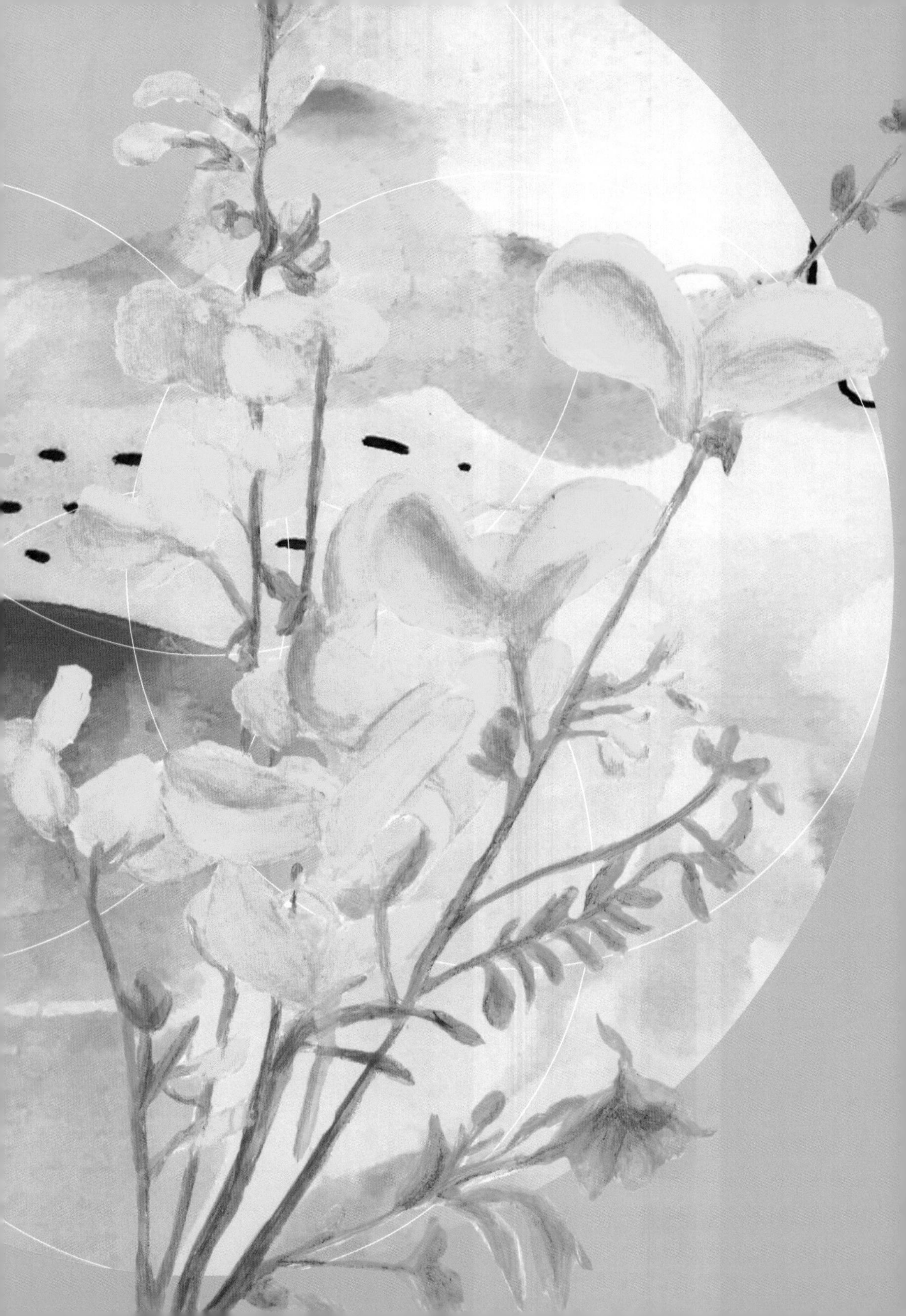

4 Flower Essences for the Blues

“

Sadness gives depth. Happiness gives height. Sadness gives roots. Happiness gives branches. Happiness is like a tree going into the sky, and sadness is like the roots going down into the womb of the earth. Both are needed, and the higher a tree goes, the deeper it goes, simultaneously. The bigger the tree, the bigger will be its roots. In fact, it is always in proportion. That's its balance.

— Osho Rajneesh

Experiencing sadness, loss, and grief is an integral part of the human experience. It is natural for the blues to get ahold of us at times. It can be an important part of how we deepen and grow as human beings. When the blanket of sadness wraps itself around you, don't push it away. Sometimes the only way out is to feel and understand your way through a complete experience. Be mindful not to grip onto the sorrow either; let the feeling move inside of you like passing clouds. Remember to always reach out and ask for the support you need. A gift of our times is that there are countless resources for when we are depressed or suffering. Never be afraid to reach out to close ones and professionals to ask for help. There is no shame in doing that—it takes strength and courage. Your peace of mind is worth it. The following flower essences also can help support you during bluesy or sad times. Sometimes the only way out is through.

Blazing Star

BLAZING STAR FLOWER ESSENCE WILL ASSIST YOU WITH:

- Healing overly emotional states
- Uniting the masculine and feminine within
- Stabilizing the spirit within

Invocation

Find a quiet spot near a fire or large rock and sit down. Meditate on your emotional body within and take Blazing Star flower essence. Then envision your sad emotions evening out like the sunset or scattered clouds across the sky. Breathe in this equanimity, knowing that you are held in a place of clarity and balance.

A purple wildflower native to the eastern United States, Blazing Star often grows in meadows. This flower essence helps lift overwrought emotional or bluesy states. After taking this essence, the fiery strength of the masculine and watery calmness of the feminine can find harmony. An inner radiance and shine may be more easily present in one's aura. This flower essence assists when one is feeling weak or frozen in emotions; it helps an individual find power again but from a place of integration.

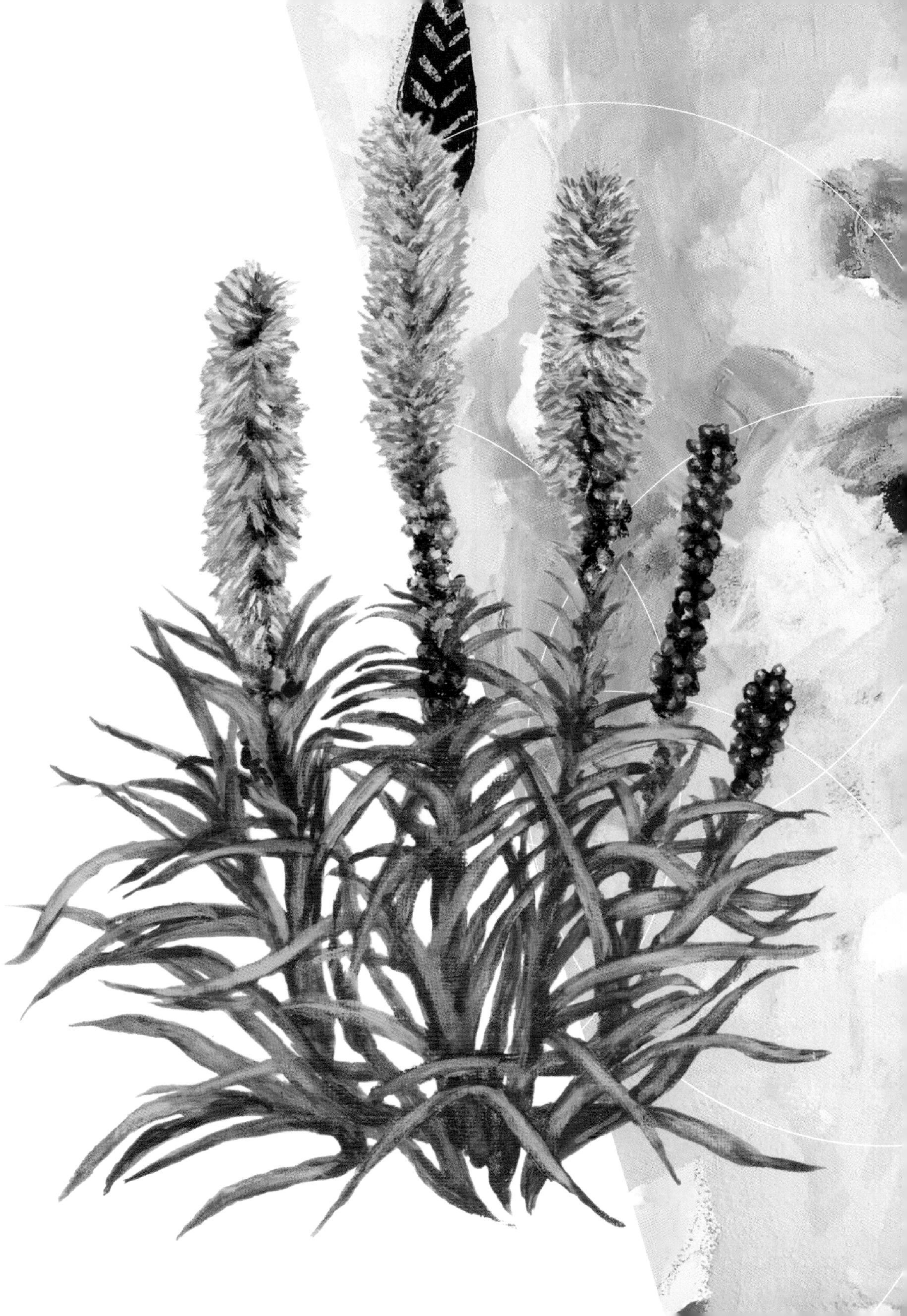

Baby Blue Eyes

BABY BLUE EYES FLOWER ESSENCE WILL ASSIST YOU WITH:

- Releasing insecurity and mistrust
- Restoring faith in spirit and a sense of belonging
- Alleviating feelings of disconnection

Invocation

Take this flower essence as you sit down under a large tree, or if inside, wrap yourself in a warm fuzzy blanket. Feel the healing effect of Baby Blue Eyes moving through you, providing you with a deep sense of connection and security in this world. Know how loved you are, despite everything you have gone through, and feel the positive effects that it inspires from within.

Found in the western part of the United States, this sweet flower grows in a variety of habitats, including grasslands and coastal bluffs. The flower essence of Baby Blue Eyes is one that provides feelings of belonging and safety and helps lift a gloomy or disconnected attitude toward life. This powerful little healer is especially appropriate for those who had a challenging childhood in relation to the father. If the father figure did not provide enough of a loving presence or sense of security to the child, the child may have a sense of vulnerability and take on a negative disposition toward the world. The result of this is feeling that one does not belong or that humans are not to be trusted. Baby Blue Eyes assists in alleviating such feelings and uplifts the soul to feel more faith and belonging. A firmer sense of trust may take root from within, thus heartening a clearer connection to spirit and higher consciousness. Let this flower essence show you that you do indeed belong and are an integral part of this world, one where you can enjoy life and feel connected to all.

Buttercup

BUTTERCUP FLOWER ESSENCE WILL ASSIST YOU WITH:

- Letting go of insecurity
- Recognizing your inner radiance and worth
- Releasing the need for external validation

Invocation

Gently cup your Buttercup flower essence in your hands. Look into a mirror, directly into your eyes, and say, "I see you and love you deeply for all that you are right now." This flower essence helps you see your true light in a simple and clear way.

Native to the western part of the United States and Canada, this yellow flower often can be found in open meadows and on forest floors. Buttercup flower essence helps souls find peace with where they are in life, especially if it's a phase in which they are feeling insecure, sad, or of low self-worth. After taking this essence, they may realize that their radiance is a true gift, no matter the outward circumstances or appearances. The inner light that one possesses can help transcend feelings of low self-worth. From this deeper realization, a quiet confidence can build, one that stops judging oneself in comparison to the standards of society, but rather is complete in its own light and truth. Buttercup gently blesses us by allowing that light to shine freely and naturally from within.

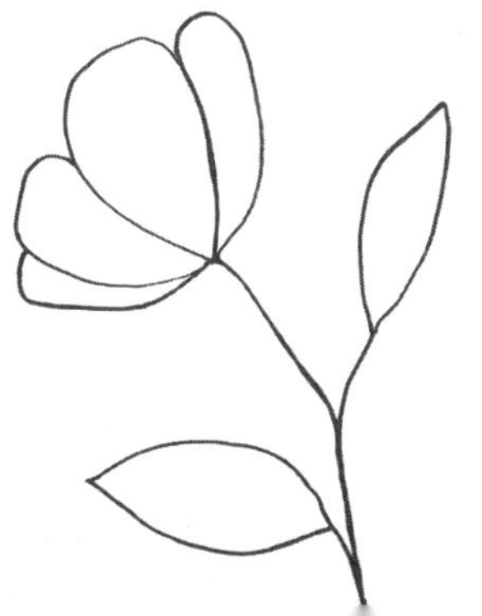

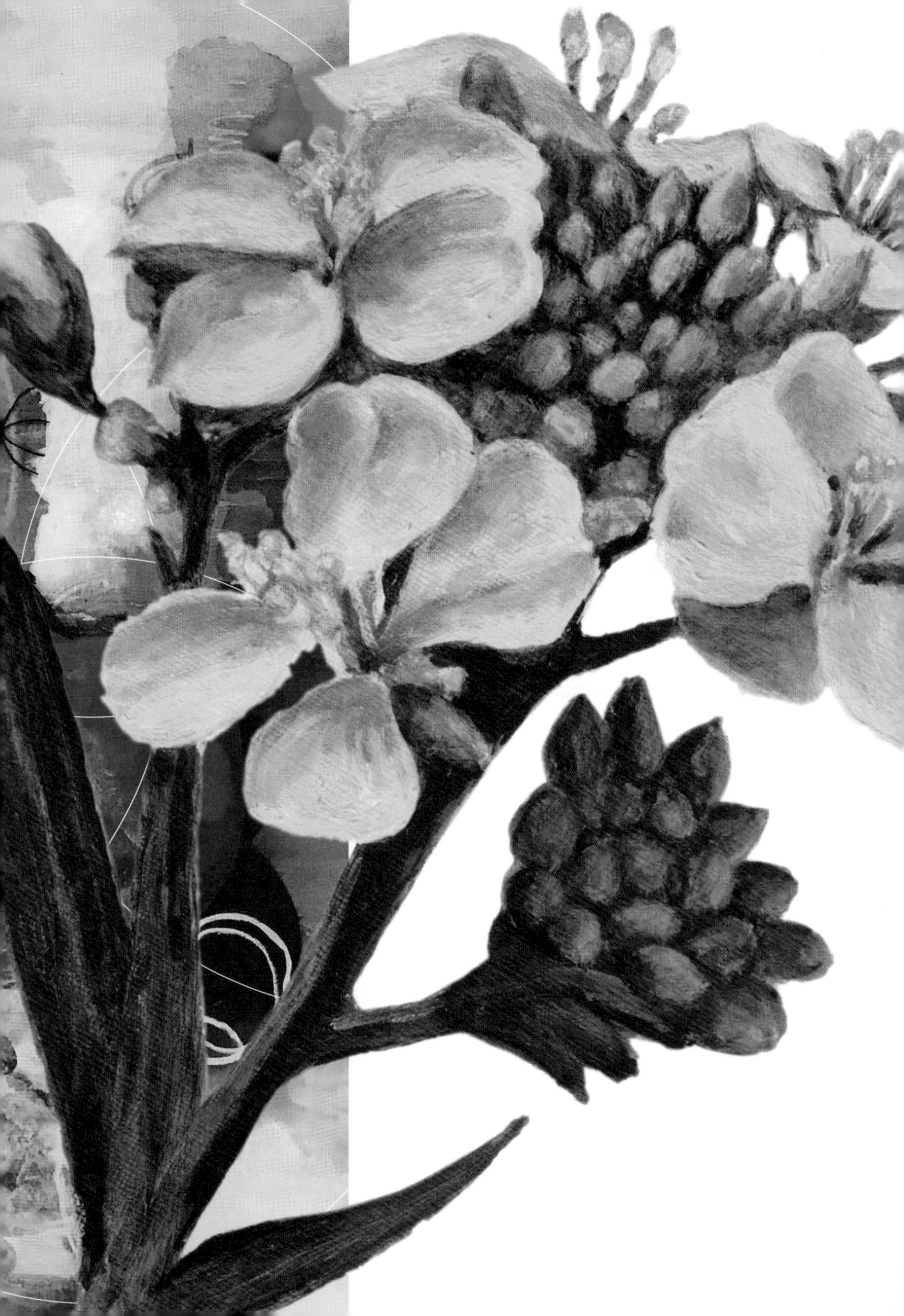

Mustard

MUSTARD FLOWER ESSENCE WILL ASSIST YOU WITH:

- Lifting depression or melancholy
- Providing support in dark times when healing is needed
- Restoring joy and gentleness

Invocation

Take this gentle yet potent healer when you are ready to reconcile events of your past to feel more at peace with today. After you take Mustard flower essence, light some candles, burn incense, and freewrite in your journal. See what comes through your hands; it may be longing to be recognized so it can be integrated and released. Allow Mustard to help you transform back to equanimity.

Also known as Wild Mustard, Charlock, or Field Mustard, this yellow-flowered plant is native to North Africa, Europe, and Asia. Mustard flower essence is an important healer for those who are feeling depressed but are unable to pinpoint why. Perhaps an accumulation of events led the soul to feel overwhelmed and in despair. This flower essence helps people recover parts of their subconscious so understanding and emotional integration can take place, thus facilitating transformation for healing. The darkness is an integral part of healing, but harmony and balance can be restored and radiance can shine again from the heart. This flower essence is a powerful tool for gaining true knowledge and liberation from the past so that peace and ease can be more of a daily part of life.

Scotch Broom

SCOTCH BROOM FLOWER ESSENCE WILL ASSIST YOU WITH:

- Healing feelings of depression and negativity
- Opening perception to more positive feelings
- Becoming more empathetic and full of purpose

Invocation

Take this flower essence into a busy part of your town or city. Sit at a café and observe the world go by. Notice your perceptions and judgments that arise. Now take Scotch Broom flower essence and sit quietly with a cup of tea. Allow new feelings to emerge from this state. Viewing the world with new eyes of compassion can help make it a better place. You are an important part of humanity's evolution.

This perennial shrub, native to parts of Europe, has golden yellow flowers that bloom plentifully in the spring and summer. Scotch Broom flower essence helps those who feel depressed and pessimistic about the challenging occurrences and news of the world. It helps alleviate feelings of uncertainty and despair so an individual may become more of an integral part of things. It also assists in shifting perception so that one can become full of radiance and purpose, glowing with compassion for the needs of others and thus humanity at large. This powerful healer allows us to meet the intensity of today's times with a motivated and more hopeful spirit. From this place, one can help those in need and inspire others with an encouraged and transformed outlook. Take Scotch Broom if you would benefit from any of these aspects and wish to make a difference, starting from within.

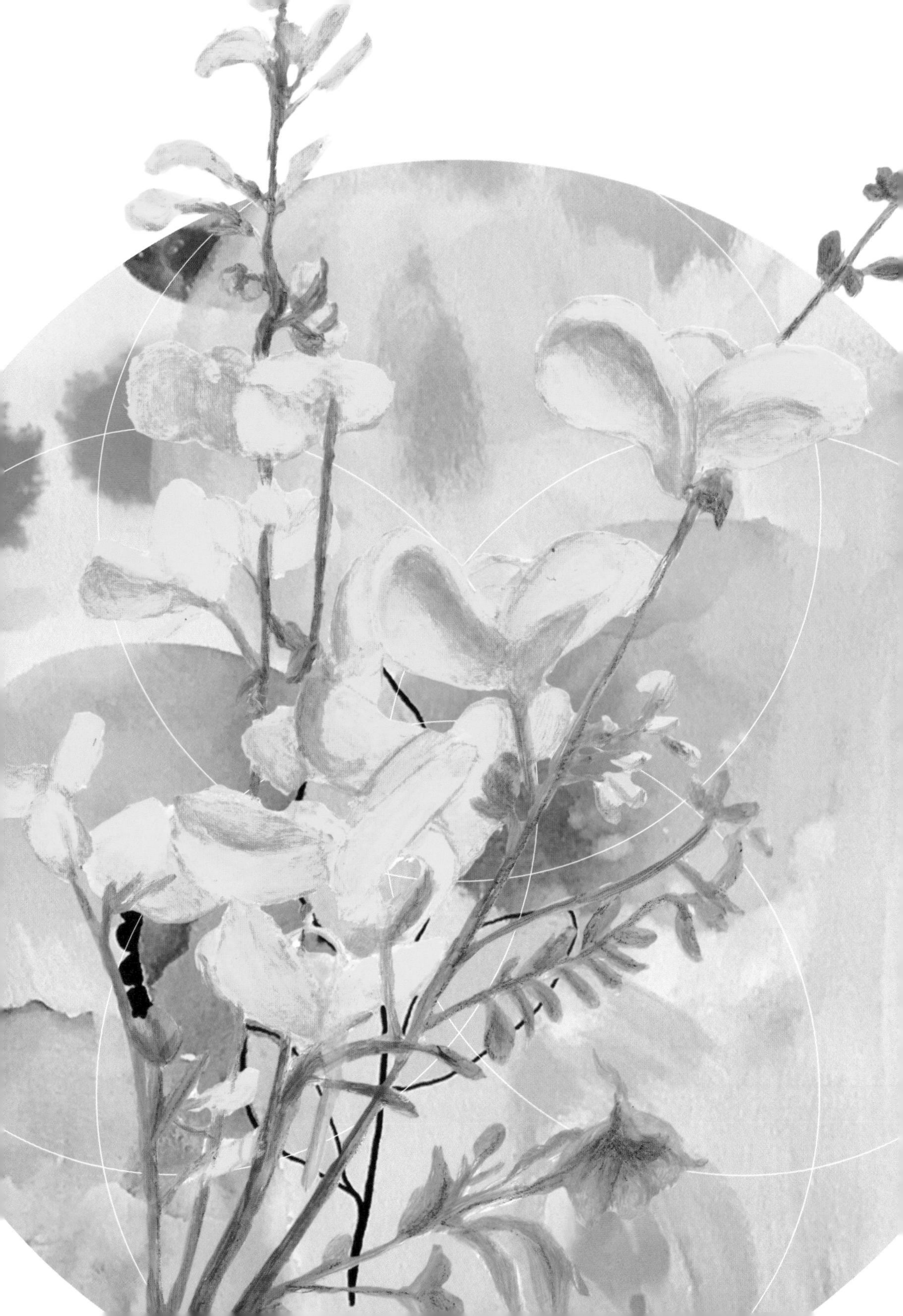

Saint John's Wort

SAINT JOHN'S WORT FLOWER ESSENCE WILL ASSIST YOU WITH:

- Healing intense fears
- Feeling protected, strong, and grounded
- Establishing light-filled awareness

Invocation

Sit before a fire, if you can, and wrap a warm blanket around you. Take this essence and envision light entering your being in a way that grounds and connects you to the earth. Know that Saint John's Wort is working its magick to help integrate and strengthen your spirit.

A yellow-flowering plant that also has herbal medicinal uses, this perennial is native to temperate parts of Asia and Europe. Saint John's Wort flower essence helps souls who have expanded their consciousness too vastly and quickly without proper integration and connection to the lower chakras. Highly sensitive souls who are allergic to environmental stress may also benefit from this flower essence. Saint John's Wort is highly restorative and provides inner fortitude and protection. It holds the body in light and helps all the chakras and layers of the field be brought back into wholeness. Those who take this potent healer go from astral projecting and "leaving the body" to experiencing light consciousness and awareness while being anchored to the earth.

Willow

WILLOW FLOWER ESSENCE WILL ASSIST YOU WITH:

- Shifting out of victim consciousness
- Finding forgiveness
- Taking ownership of your life

Invocation

Take this flower essence and then grab your journal. Make a list of people you need to forgive. If it feels good to you, write about ways in which you have grown and learned from the experiences they've given you. Burn that piece of paper or bury it in the earth. Realize this: You truly are the captain of your own ship. Let the sailing go more smoothly now as you find your own flow and grace once again.

A large deciduous tree native to Asia and Europe, Willow has a fast growth rate and pale leaves. Willow flower essence brings about many gifts for a soul who is stuck feeling like a victim of life. The healing qualities of this essence shine forth acceptance and taking ownership of one's life, so life can flow in a state of natural ease. Being able to forgive more freely is also a valuable quality of this essence. It can also shift feelings of resentment and bitterness so that they start to subside. Allow your being to step into owning your worth and take the reins of your life into your own hands. Find an inner strength within. This may feel new and a bit scary at first, but it is worth it. You are worth this state of sovereign grace.

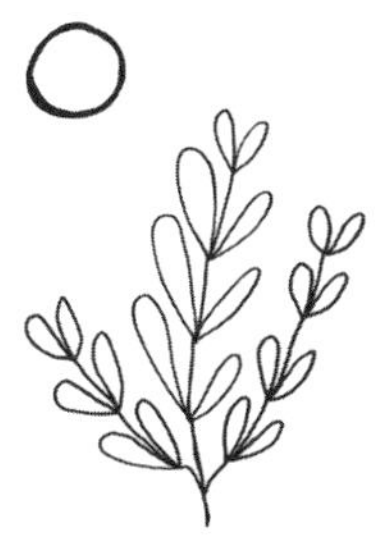

Yerba Santa

YERBA SANTA FLOWER ESSENCE WILL ASSIST YOU WITH:

- Releasing internalized grief
- Allowing emotions to flow
- Connecting more deeply to the breath

Invocation

Find a body of water such as a river, pond, lake, or ocean. Sit and notice how the light reflects on it as it moves. Take this flower essence and connect to your breath, allowing your heart chakra or chest area to open. Cry if you need to cry; let your emotions bubble out like that water. We can find harmony when our repressed energetic imprints are released and we can flow again. Feel the expansion and blessing this essence brings into your being.

Also known as the sacred or holy herb, this aromatic evergreen shrub with violet flowers is native to California and Oregon in the western United States. This flower essence helps free up repressed emotions, such as internalized sorrow or depression in the most sensitive part of the heart chakra. Yerba Santa will help inspire more life force, particularly the breath, to flow there and free up those stagnant areas. After taking this essence, one should draw attention to the breath and direct it to feelings of tightness in the chest. By making this a daily practice until one notices a shift and feels all feelings again, the individual allows the heart space to be filled with presence, a free-flowing grace that is here in the now.

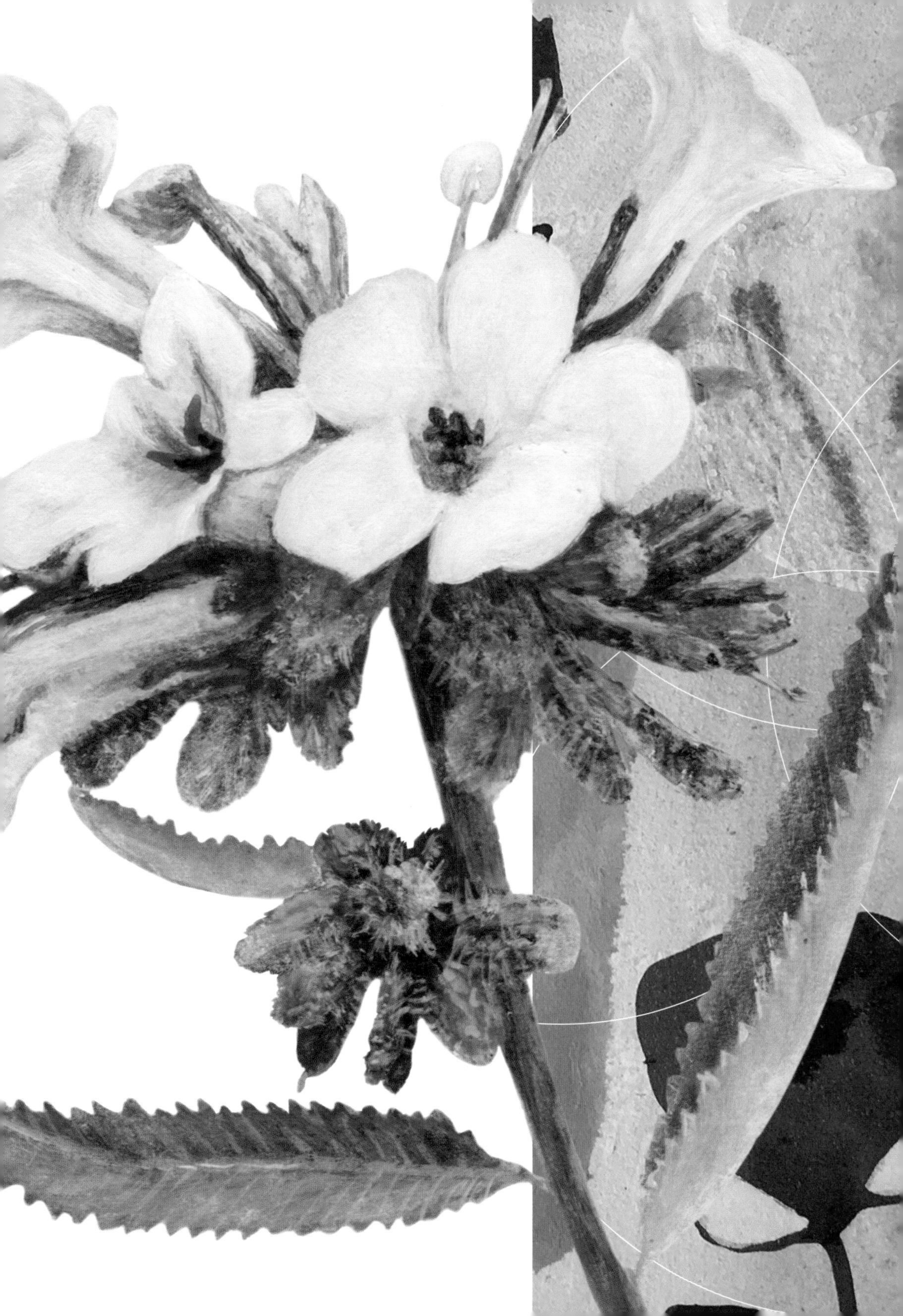

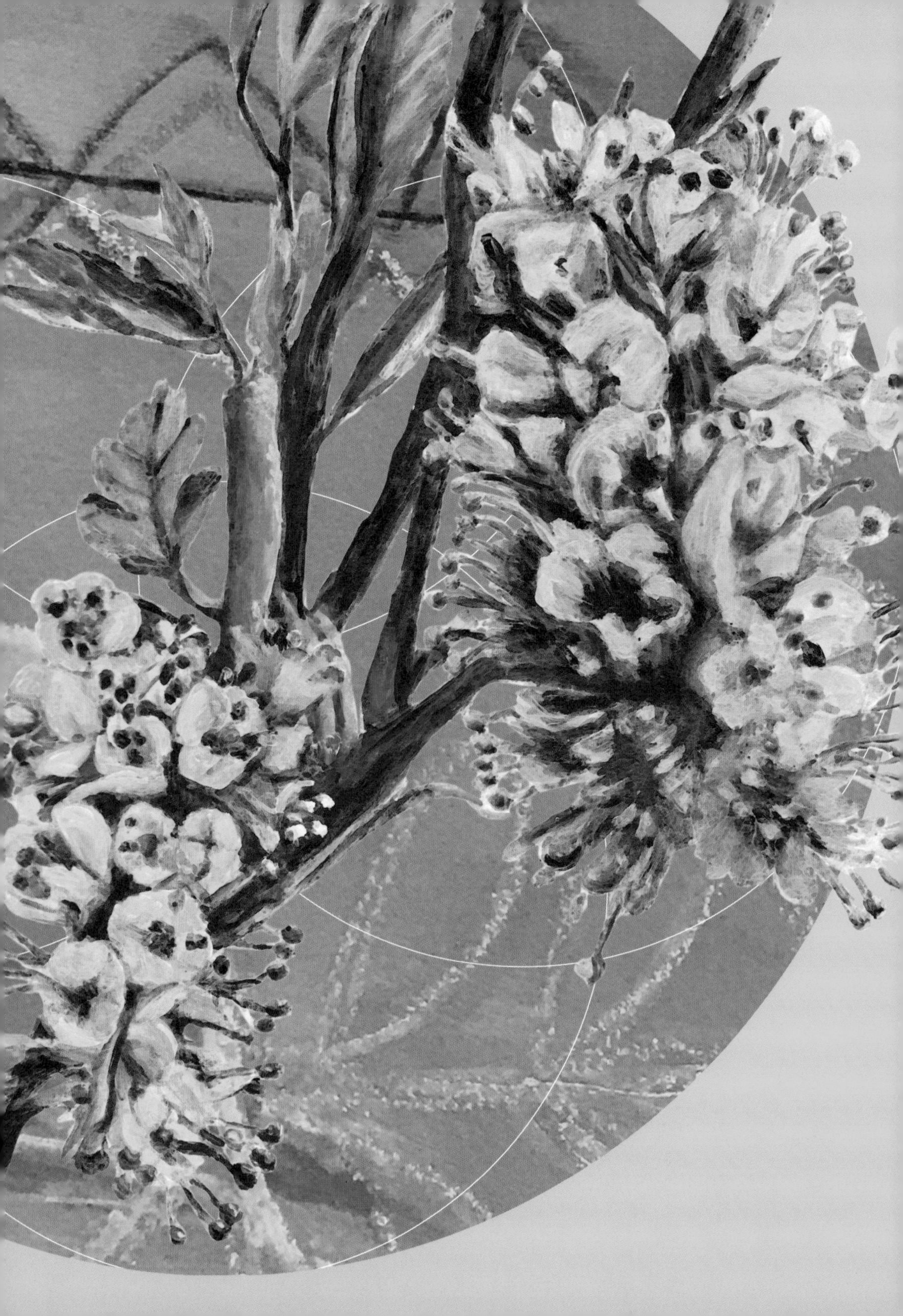

5 Flower Essences for Boundaries

If you want to live an authentic, meaningful life, you need to master the art of disappointing and upsetting others, hurting feelings, and living with the reality that some people just won't like you. It may not be easy, but it's essential if you want your life to reflect your deepest desires, values, and needs.

— Cheryl Richardson

An art professor once explained to me that our creativity can flourish more easily when we have boundaries or some structure when facing a blank canvas. He meant that boundaries help tell us where we can go and where we can't. They help us feel clarity when making decisions for ourselves. Boundaries allow us to feel safer and, in a way, more liberated! Boundaries and knowing the limits are essential for living a life through the heart. With them, we can give freely but know where our internal *yes* and *no* lies. This helps create respect and trust in all our relationships and helps us show up more authentically for others and ourselves. If we are constantly trying to please other people while neglecting our own needs, we can become resentful. Resentment is a toxic emotion that can undermine relationships. Know your *yes* and know your *no*. Allow healthy boundaries to create an enriched garden within your own internal landscape. The flower essences in this chapter can help heal any people-pleasing issues you might have and establish boundaries that allow your relationships (including the most important one, the one with yourself) to flourish.

Agrimony

AGRIMONY FLOWER ESSENCE WILL ASSIST YOU WITH:

- Attaining inner peace
- Being truthful about your real feelings
- Releasing perfectionism

Invocation

Take this flower essence before having an important talk with a loved one. Say a mantra to yourself regarding the value of honesty about emotions and feelings, such as "My true feelings matter and need to be heard." Agrimony flower essence helps dispel any denial of authentic feelings and allows honest vulnerability to come forth.

The five-petal yellow flowers of Agrimony bloom from June to September and can reach up to a height of 40 inches (1 m). Native to England and Scotland, this flower has a rich folkloric history as a magical medicinal herb. The flower essence, however, is helpful for people who struggle with always putting on a happy face no matter what they are feeling or experiencing. You would benefit from taking Agrimony if you cover up and repress suffering and instead mask it with a cheery disposition. Maintaining healthy boundaries with others can often be an issue as well because your true feelings are often hidden. Agrimony can help release the societal or familial conditioning to always have a polite attitude no matter what is going on. You may also benefit from taking this essence if you constantly seek external validation. Let Agrimony provide true peace and integration within for the whole self, not just the parts you think others want to see.

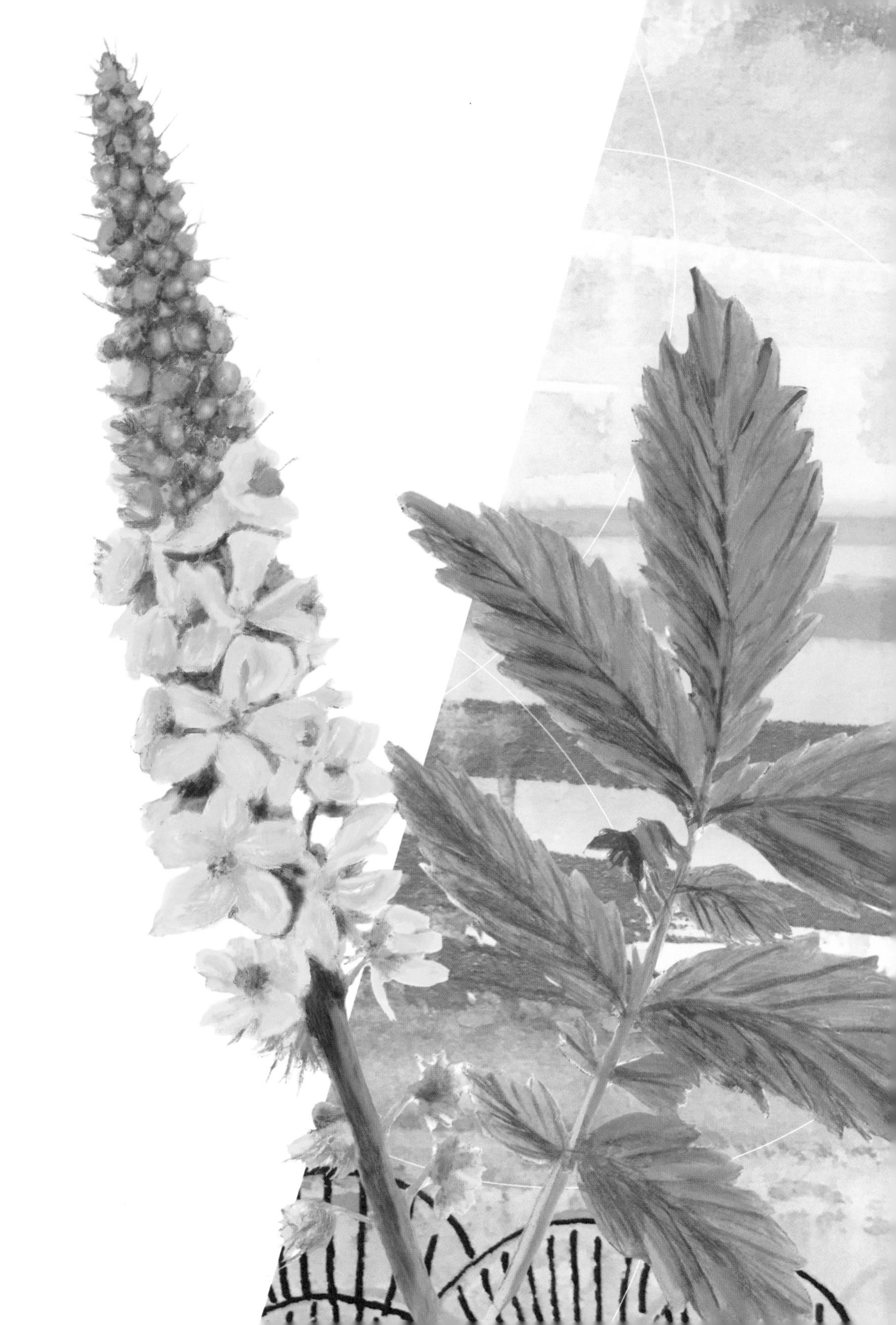

Black Cohosh

BLACK COHOSH FLOWER ESSENCE WILL ASSIST YOU WITH:

- Establishing boundaries in toxic relationships
- Breaking patterns of destructive behavior
- Transforming fear into power

Invocation

Take out your journal and write about your definition of a healthy, sustainable relationship. What qualities need to be there? Write down ways in which boundaries are naturally respected. What boundaries have you set for yourself and others? How can you improve or implement more boundaries for a healthy bond? Black Cohosh is here to support you in creating loving, respectful relationships that last.

Native to eastern regions of North America and varying parts of the Midwest, this flowering plant is best known for its medicinal properties, which have long been used by Native Americans. This powerful flower essence is helpful for people who are caught in addictive and abusive patterns, especially in relationships. You may benefit from taking Black Cohosh if you have a magnetic aura that attracts many souls looking for healing. Abusive and obsessive relationships can then manifest. This flower essence helps break patterns of attracting and being attracted to toxic relationships or trauma-bonding dynamics. By taking Black Cohosh, you may find yourself regaining new power and harmony within yourself, thereby establishing healthy boundaries and attracting a partner who can truly meet you.

Centaury

CENTAURY FLOWER ESSENCE WILL ASSIST YOU WITH:

- Building inner strength
- Releasing people-pleasing patterns
- Taking care of your needs

Invocation

Say this mantra out loud to yourself five times: "No is a complete sentence." Then take the Centaury flower essence, knowing that your needs for a healthy relationship—not only with others but also with yourself—come first.

Blooming from June to September, this pink-flowered plant is native to many parts of Europe, northern Africa, and western Asia. The Centaury flower essence is appropriate for those who find themselves feeling unable to tell others "no" and thus neglect their own needs. To serve others with ease, one needs to have a whole self to fall back on; this way, feelings of resentment and depletion won't come up later. The need for constant external validation is a shadow side of the soul that would benefit from taking Centaury. By taking this essence, one will gain inner resolve and fortitude to understand one's own boundaries and needs, and, in return, one will be able to show up more authentically for others.

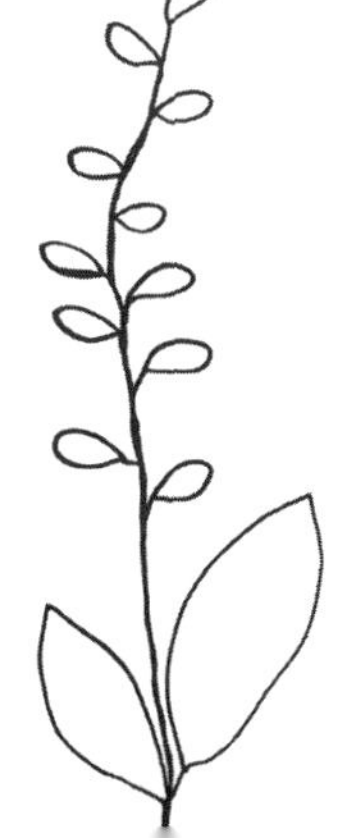

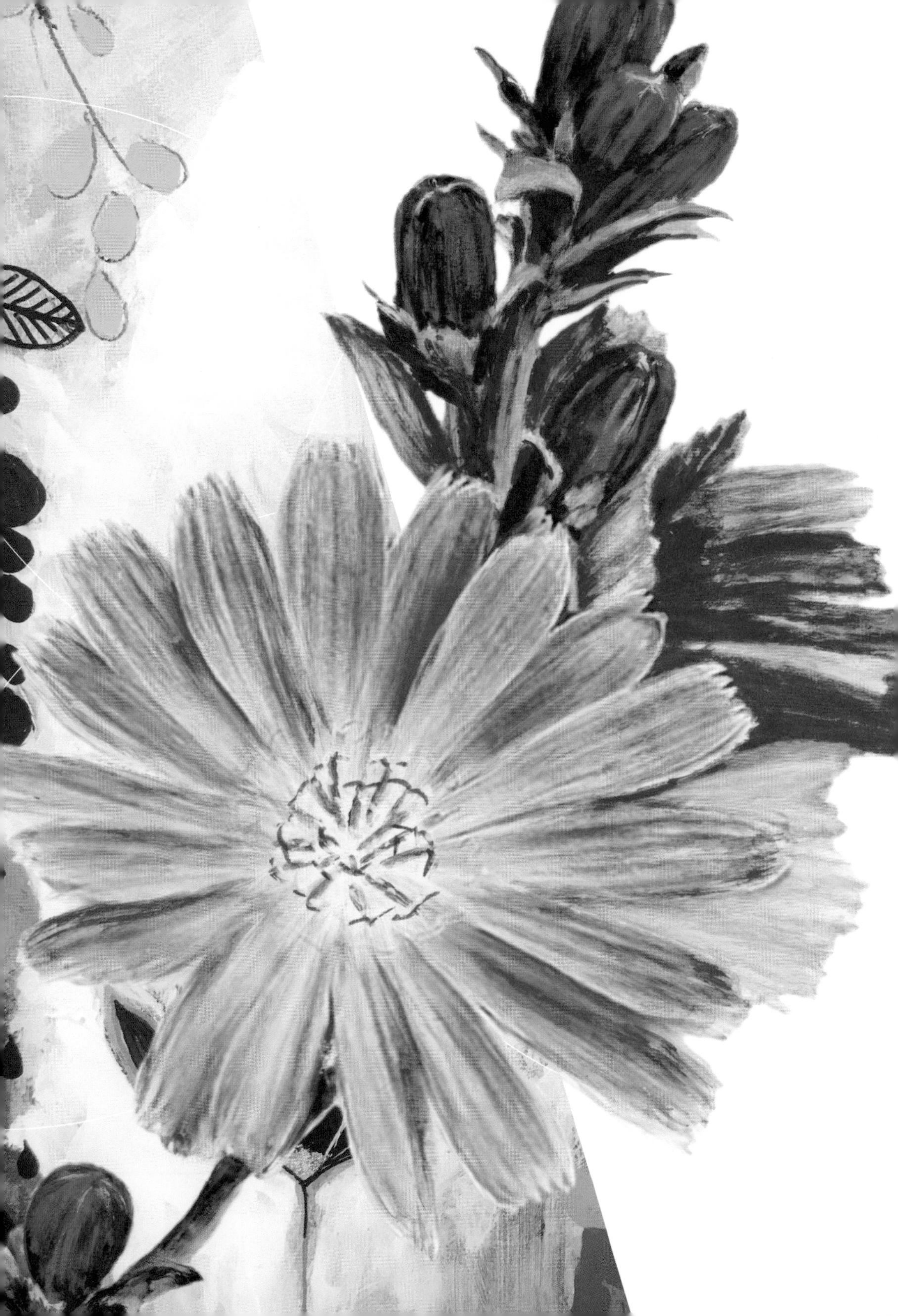

Chicory

CHICORY FLOWER ESSENCE WILL ASSIST YOU WITH:

- Respecting others' boundaries
- Giving love freely without expectations
- Releasing manipulative tendencies

Invocation

Take this flower essence and then perform random acts of kindness for others, with no expectation and with no one else seeing or hearing about it. Chicory bestows the gift of selflessness in its highest form. Reap the benefits of this essence and free yourself from possessive and manipulative energy.

Native to Europe, this perennial plant belongs to the dandelion family. It has bright blue flowers and the leaves are often used in salads or other edibles. Someone who becomes possessive in love and selfish in intention would benefit from taking Chicory. In relationships, if you find yourself manipulating your partner's emotions so your own needs can be met, consider taking this flower essence. In truth, these behaviors can be a form of neediness disguised as love, and neediness and love are two different things. Chicory flower essence assists in healing such negative patterns and establishing healthy boundaries. Energy can begin to flow from the heart in a more unconditional way, thus transforming the bond into a mutually authentic loving relationship.

Oak

OAK FLOWER ESSENCE WILL ASSIST YOU WITH:

- Enveloping strength during great challenge
- Learning to rest and restore
- Embracing surrender

Invocation

Take Oak flower essence with you outside and lie down on a blanket. After consuming the flower essence, envision your energy completely letting go, allowing Mother Earth to take care of the stress. Breathe deep into all your cells and feel the release that this rest brings. Trust that in order to overcome great challenges, you must also learn the art of surrender.

Native to the Americas, Asia, Europe, and North Africa, the Oak tree or shrub has approximately 600 species in the genus *Quercus*. Oak flower essence is best known for helping people who are relentless in their determination and who can be downright inflexible at times. If you often find yourself working beyond your limit and taking on more than you can handle emotionally, physically, or mentally, this flower essence can help. Oak helps bring about balance to such a strong will, along with respecting and knowing one's limits. It may inspire self-care and rest when one begins to feel overworked. The gift of the Oak flower essence is the art of surrender, which allows energy to naturally flow that aligns with the universe or source energy. Take this essence if you wish to learn the gift of knowing when to let go and slow down.

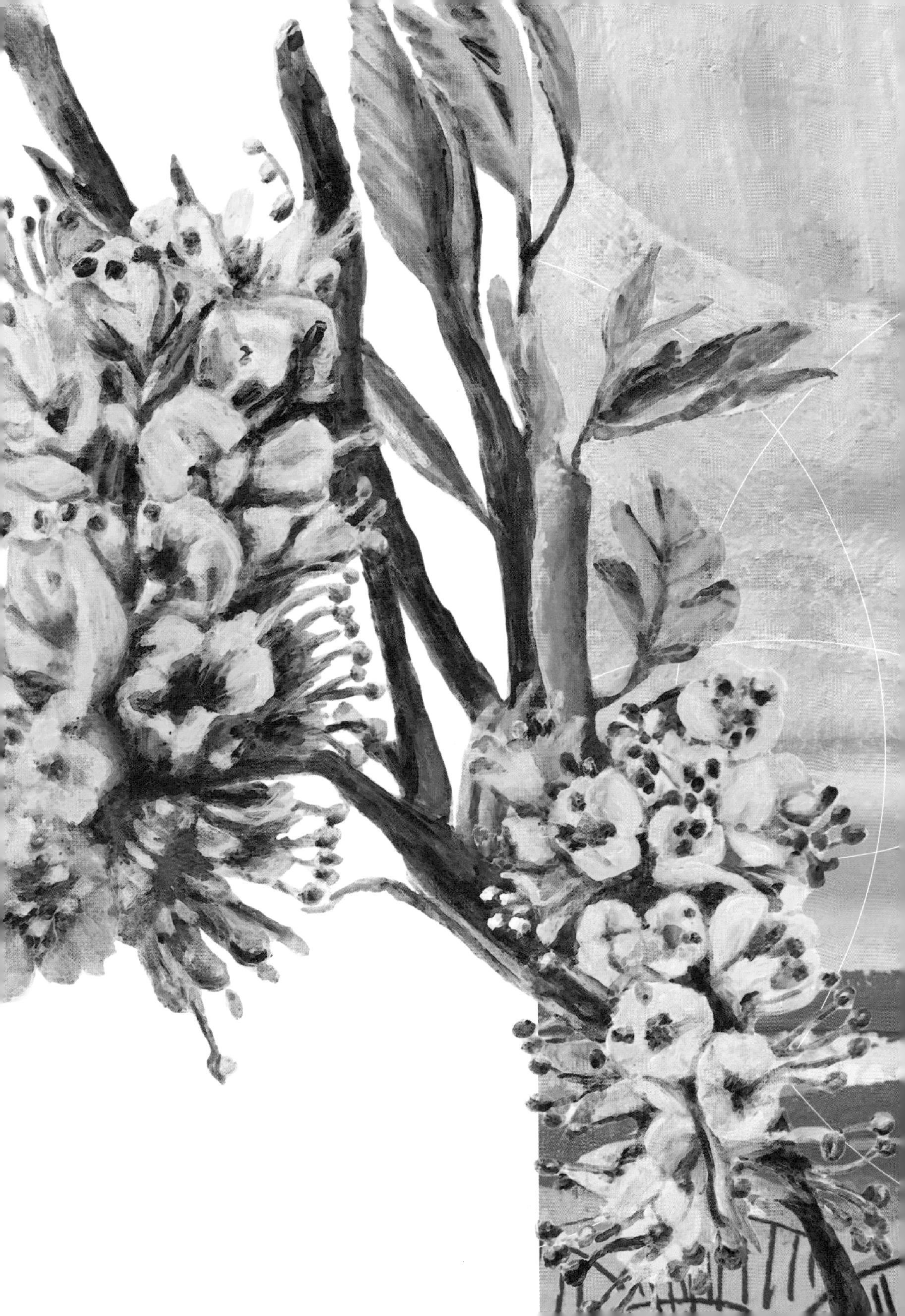

Quince

QUINCE FLOWER ESSENCE WILL ASSIST YOU WITH:

- Integrating the masculine and feminine within
- Understanding that real love empowers
- Balancing aspects of giving love

Invocation

Hold the Quince flower essence in your hands and say this mantra out loud: "I honor the soft feminine and powerful masculine within me. I know both are an integral part of my being. I can love freely with gentleness and strength." After taking Quince, see how your relationships evolve in the flow of both giving and receiving.

Native to Asia, this red flower is a deciduous shrub that is known for its medicinal properties in Chinese medicine. Quince flower essence provides a harmonious relationship with both the masculine and the feminine. It brings about integration so that loving in a powerful yet gentle way is easily possible for both women and men. As a result, clearer boundaries can be established, and one will know when more feminine or masculine aspects are needed when sharing space or giving love to someone special. Love shouldn't compromise us, but it can soften us with its inherent force alone. Quince demonstrates that love is an energy that empowers effortlessly and with grace, and those around the individual taking it can reap the benefits.

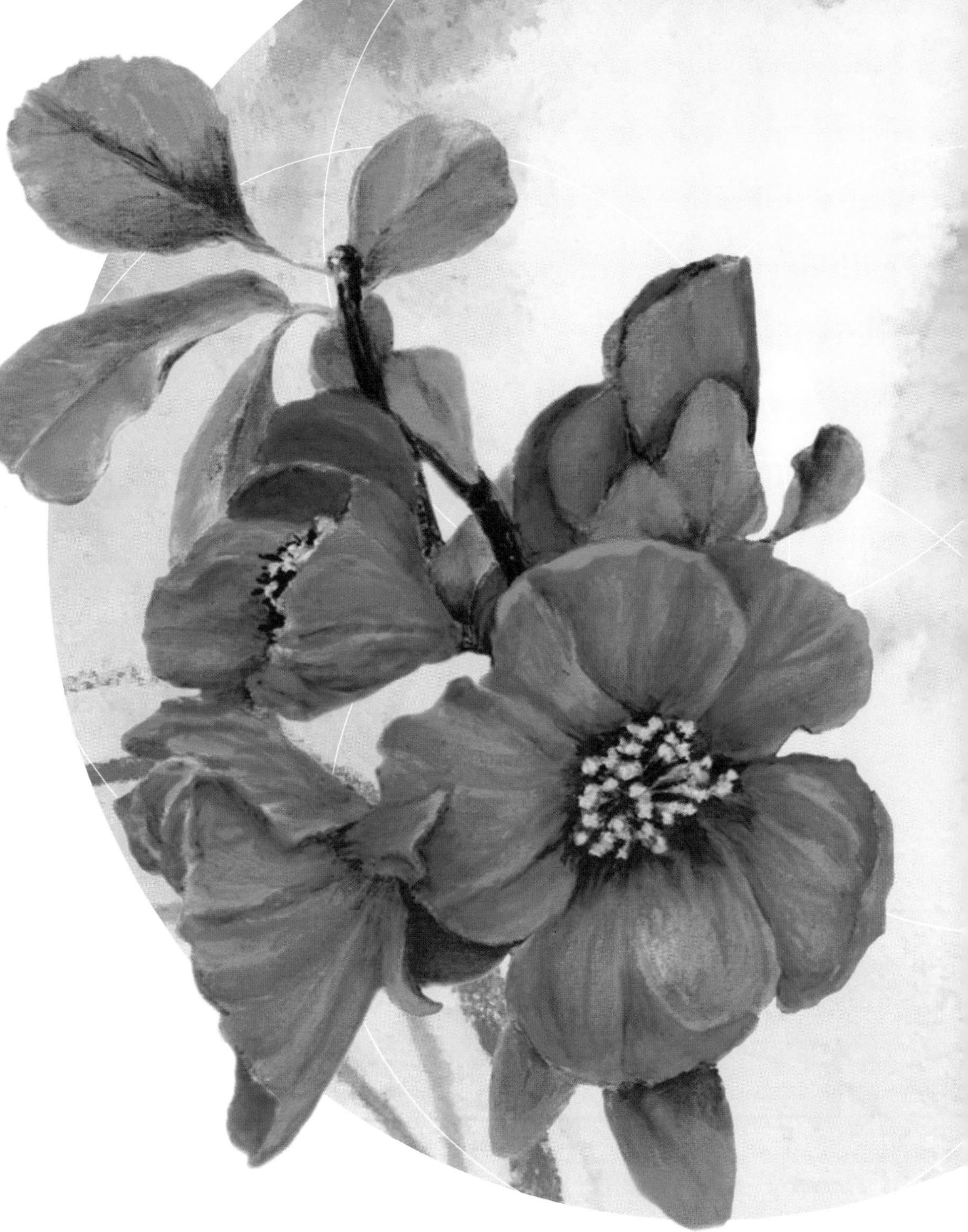

Red Chestnut

RED CHESTNUT FLOWER ESSENCE WILL ASSIST YOU WITH:

- Overcoming worry about others
- Fearfulness about upcoming events
- Feeling trust and peace within, especially in regard to others

Invocation

Before you spend time with a loved one about whom you worry, take this flower essence. Allow its healing medicine to enter your nervous system and relax you. Feel the peace it brings. Know your loved one is safe and their journey is theirs alone to take.

The origins of this hybrid tree are not specifically known, but it possibly came from Germany in the early 1800s. The Red Chestnut tree is popular as an ornamental in gardens and public parks and can grow up to 80 feet (24.4 m) tall; it blooms beautiful red flowers. The Red Chestnut flower is an apropos healer for those who overly worry and fear for others. People who are naturally drawn into the empathic caretaker role and tend to take on negative emotions of others would benefit from taking this essence. These behaviors actually can create patterns that do not allow the other soul to heal and move forward from this codependent dynamic or bondage in relationship. True integration of healing for both souls, especially the one who worries, can ground and take root when the caretaker becomes more embodied in their own self and connection to vibrant source energy. Red Chestnut offers beautiful assistance to allow the caretaker or worrier to become trusting in the lives of others and in their own peace. This flower essence can be good especially for those who offer themselves as empaths and healers in family dynamics and systems. If you find yourself persistently anxious about others' fate and life journey, allow this flower essence to bestow calm and loving presence within your field, thus greatly benefiting your soul as well as the lives of others.

Scarlet Monkeyflower

SCARLET MONKEYFLOWER FLOWER ESSENCE WILL ASSIST YOU WITH:

- Repressing intense emotions
- Communicating clearly and honestly
- Becoming aware of your shadow

Invocation

Take this flower essence before you sit down to meditate or write. Allow it to reveal your true feelings within, especially ones that are more charged with negative emotions. Now sit and breathe and notice those emotions; let yourself become more fully aware of them. You may also wish to write down these feelings in detail. Let your emotions flow freely and make a pact to become more honest with others about what you really feel.

Native to the West Coast of the United States, this flowering perennial with red-orange blossoms is widely cultivated as an ornamental plant. Its luscious large blooms with ample nectar attract hummingbirds. The flower essence of Scarlet Monkeyflower is a potent healer for those who have trouble establishing honest and consistent communication about their real feelings. If you struggle to be direct about charged or negative emotions, this essence could be beneficial for you. Scarlet Monkeyflower assists in uncovering repressed emotions and attaining awareness of the shadow self. For instance, if these emotions do not integrate within the conscious self, you may find yourself exploding with rage or raw emotions due to lack of communication and healthy boundaries. If you notice this is a pattern for you, let Scarlet Monkeyflower bestow its blessing onto you, providing clarity and truth-telling in relationship to others. This will allow for fullness of spirit and authentic relating within yourself, thus inspiring wholeheartedness in all your relations.

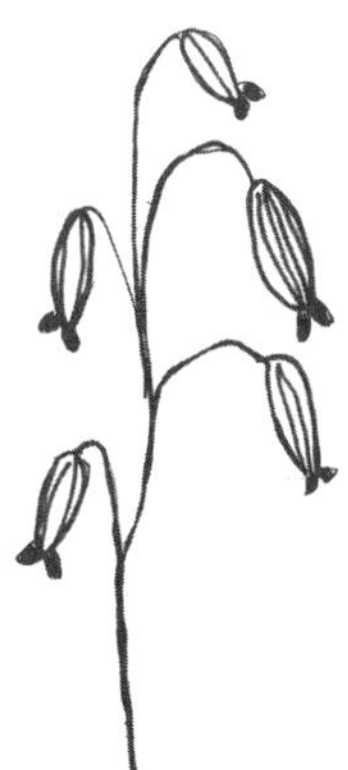

6 Flower Essences for a Broken Heart

"

Life will break you. Nobody can protect you from that, and living alone won't either, for solitude will also break you with its yearning. You have to love. You have to feel. It is the reason you are here on earth. You are here to risk your heart. You are here to be swallowed up. And when it happens that you are broken, or betrayed, or left, or hurt, or death brushes near, let yourself sit by an apple tree and listen to the apples falling all around you in heaps, wasting their sweetness. Tell yourself you tasted as many as you could.

— Louise Erdrich

The absolute hardest times in life can come when we experience a broken heart. Oh, the intense pain and heartache—it can feel so unbearable and confusing. Perhaps, though, a broken heart is an initiation into a life that is more truthful and aligned with purpose. Perhaps through the tears and grief, one can find true strength and solace within. It is in that grief that a clearer mind and sovereign soul can emerge. From that place, a more honest and happier life—one that is in alignment with your true self—can emerge. You can learn vast amounts about yourself and others during times of strongest heartbreak. Allow your broken heart to show you the way, trust its lesson, and find strength in the new self that emerges. You will forever be changed, and that is a good thing. The flower essence formulas in this chapter can support you on this mending and healing for your heart. Take care, dear traveler, and be so very gentle with yourself.

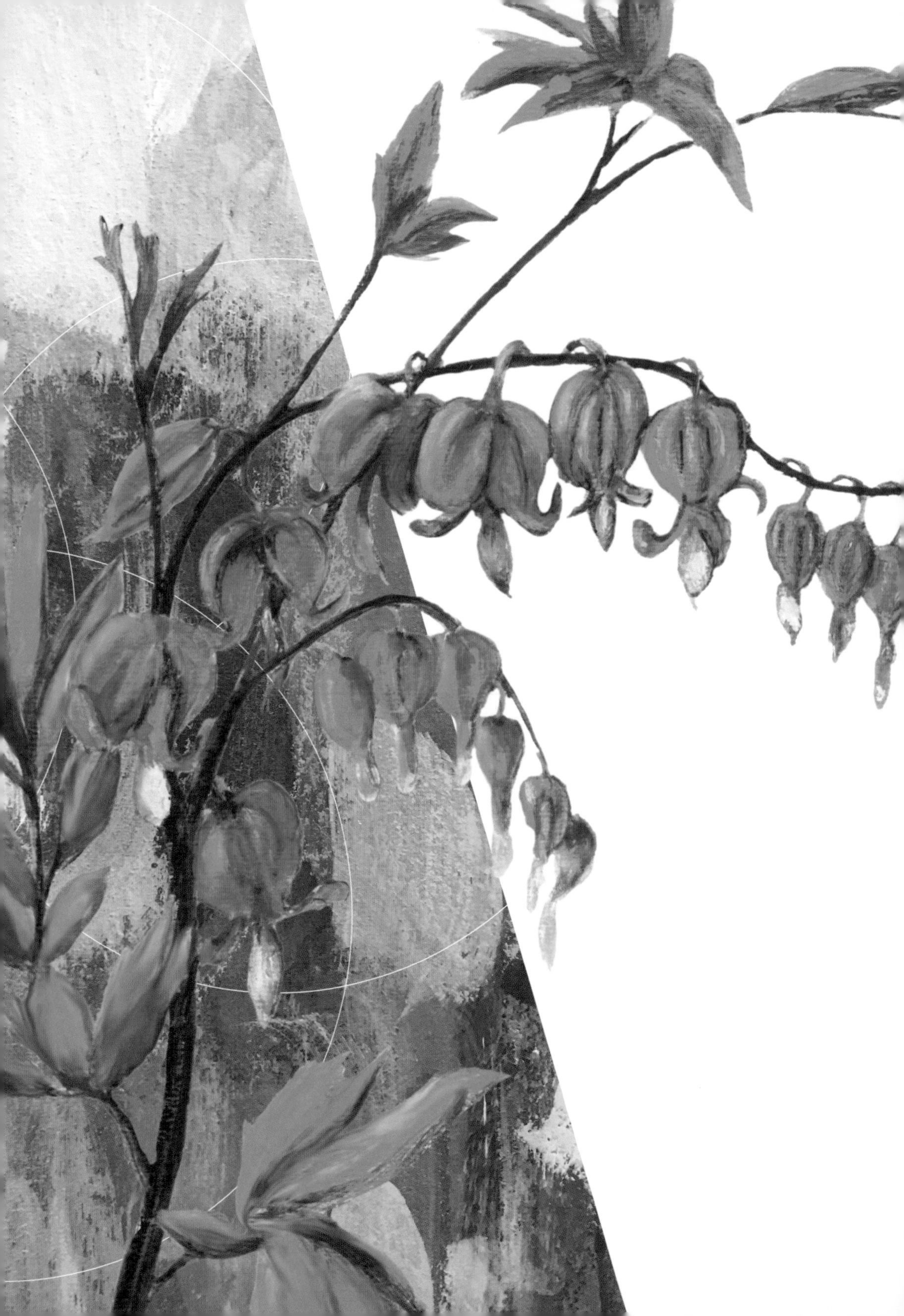

Bleeding Heart

BLEEDING HEART FLOWER ESSENCE WILL ASSIST YOU WITH:

- Letting go of codependent patterns
- Feeling emotionally free
- Forming healthy and strong loving bonds

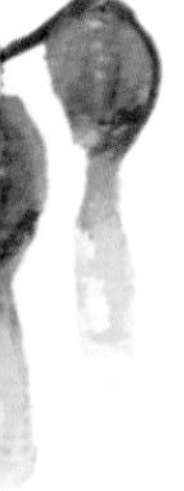

Invocation

Take this flower essence and light a candle. Place both hands on your heart and watch the flame flicker. Witness how it dances and yet remains full of life, sovereign and strong. Breathe into your hands and the energy of your heart. Hold your loving attention there and know that all will be well.

With pink, heart-shaped flowers, this perennial herbaceous plant is native to Asia. It grows in moist woodlands and forests. Bleeding Heart flower essence is for mending a broken heart due to loss of a relationship or loved one. It is appropriate for healing insecurity or codependent feelings in relationships, when you feel like you need the other person to exist and wish to possess them out of fear of loneliness. Or perhaps you have been in a relationship for a while but you have lost your sense of self due to a lack of boundaries or enabling patterns. Whatever the case, your loving heart has been overworked and compromised by loving a bit too much. The magick of Bleeding Heart essence is that it inspires you to love from a place that is unconditional and deeply connected to source energy. When love for oneself strengthens, so does the ability to give and receive love freely, and that is more satisfying for all. Consider Bleeding Heart if you have felt the desire to be needed from a place of lack or heartache and wish to give and receive love from a place that sustains and fulfills.

Borage

BORAGE FLOWER ESSENCE WILL ASSIST YOU WITH:

- Uplifting a heavy heart
- Building trust and confidence
- Heartening optimism and joy

Invocation

Rub some sweet-smelling oils on your heart and solar plexus area (right above your belly button). Take this flower essence and go on a walk, dance a little, or do something else to get you moving. Feel how you can lighten up with each step and trust the wisdom of your heart. You've got this.

Native to the Mediterranean, this flowering annual plant has a rich history of culinary and herbal medicine use. Borage flower essence is a pertinent healer for those who are feeling heavy in their heart and body. This can come naturally after a loss or a period of grief. One of the many gifts of this essence is that it inspires warmth and radiance in the human form and uplifts the energy so that it moves again from a place of source light within. Borage flower essence restores an innate sense of joy and buoyancy with hope for the future. This returned sense of optimism and courage will help you move forward and gravitate toward more experiences that will fulfill you. Let Borage work its jubilant forces inside you so that you can lift into new realms of being.

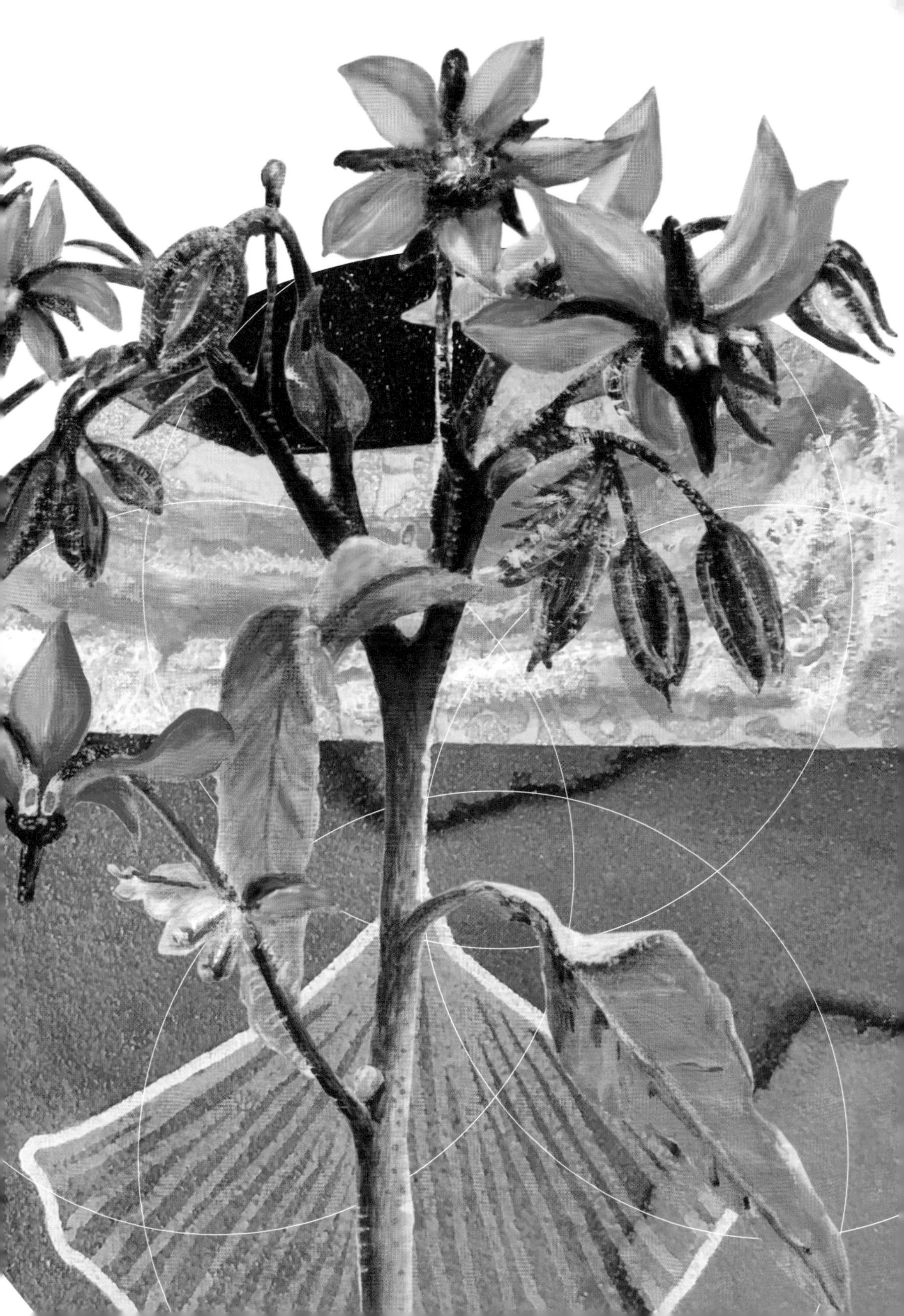

Forget-Me-Not

FORGET-ME-NOT FLOWER ESSENCE WILL ASSIST YOU WITH:

- Alleviating isolation and disconnection
- Establishing heart-based relations
- Cultivating awareness of other realms

Invocation

Create an altar space to honor loved ones who have passed, even if it's just taking out a photo of them. Take Forget-Me-Not flower essence, say a prayer of gratitude, and honor your ancestors. Feel the connection and healing this experience brings.

A flowering plant native to Europe, and since widely cultivated all over the earth, this sweet little flower blooms in a sky-blue color in the spring. The healing power of Forget-Me-Not flower essence brings about connection to other dimensions and realms, especially when tuning in to loved ones or ancestors who have passed. It also aids in alleviating feelings of isolation and disconnection here on earth and in the three-dimensional realm. Forget-Me-Not flower essence is especially opportune when dealing with grief of the loss of a loved one. It assists in keeping that connection alive in your heart and helps integrate life without your loved one here on earth. Another gift of this flower essence is that it guides you into understanding karmic relationships, both living and passed away. This insight can be incredibly beneficial for your own soul's transformation and the illumination of your path in terms of relationships.

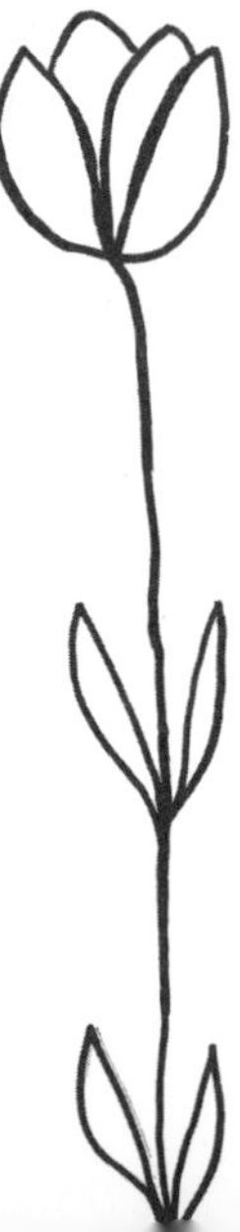

Honeysuckle

HONEYSUCKLE FLOWER ESSENCE WILL ASSIST YOU WITH:

- Easing attachment to the past
- Becoming fully present in the moment
- Understanding lessons from the past

Invocation

Take Honeysuckle flower essence and find your journal or some sheets of paper. Begin to write events of the past that you feel stuck on or that are holding you back. After freewriting from your subconscious for about ten to fifteen minutes, ask to be released from the past. You can tear these sheets up, bury them, or even burn them. Let this flower essence support you in fully living in the moment.

Native to Europe, these perennial plants are best known for their sweet and intoxicating aromas. They are active climbers, and they have tiny white flowers with highlights of red or pink that bloom in the summer. Honeysuckle flower essence is a good formula for healing people who are stuck in events and thoughts of the past and feeling overly nostalgic. When our mind lives in the past, it is easy to feel sadness or stagnation, for the presence and life source energy as it exists now cannot be felt and appreciated. Perceptions of current reality can get cloudy, and presented gifts cannot fully be acted upon. A soul can become trapped and low in vital energy without even realizing it. If you find yourself looking to the past and clinging to those emotions or experiences, the Honeysuckle flower essence is ideal for you. Live in the now and recognize the peace this brings.

Jasmine

JASMINE FLOWER ESSENCE WILL ASSIST YOU WITH:

- Healing emotional trauma from the past
- Releasing stagnation from past concepts
- Inspiring an open heart

Invocation

Wrap yourself in a comfortable robe or silky pajamas and take this flower essence. Put on some soft music and place your hands over your heart. Imagine your heart opening up to the moonlight ever so gently. Allow yourself to release stories of the past, thoughts, and ideas that no longer serve you.

A widely cultivated, highly aromatic flower, this genus of vines belongs to the olive family and is native to temperate regions of Eurasia, Australia, New Zealand, and Oceania. Jasmine flower essence is concerned with releasing energetic stuck feelings in the heart. These feelings often come from past lovers or old traumas. But this sweet healer provides a soft opening in the heart and receptivity to the power of feminine nature. It builds feelings of worthiness and belonging so that the inner alchemy can find harmony and attract love and connection that is worthy of your precious heart. It stirs us to feel unconditional love toward ourselves first, thus releasing the need for others to desire us. If you have found yourself caught in mental loops from the past, allow Jasmine's prowess to inspire you to a softening and profound love for the self. Watch how your life transforms from this awakening.

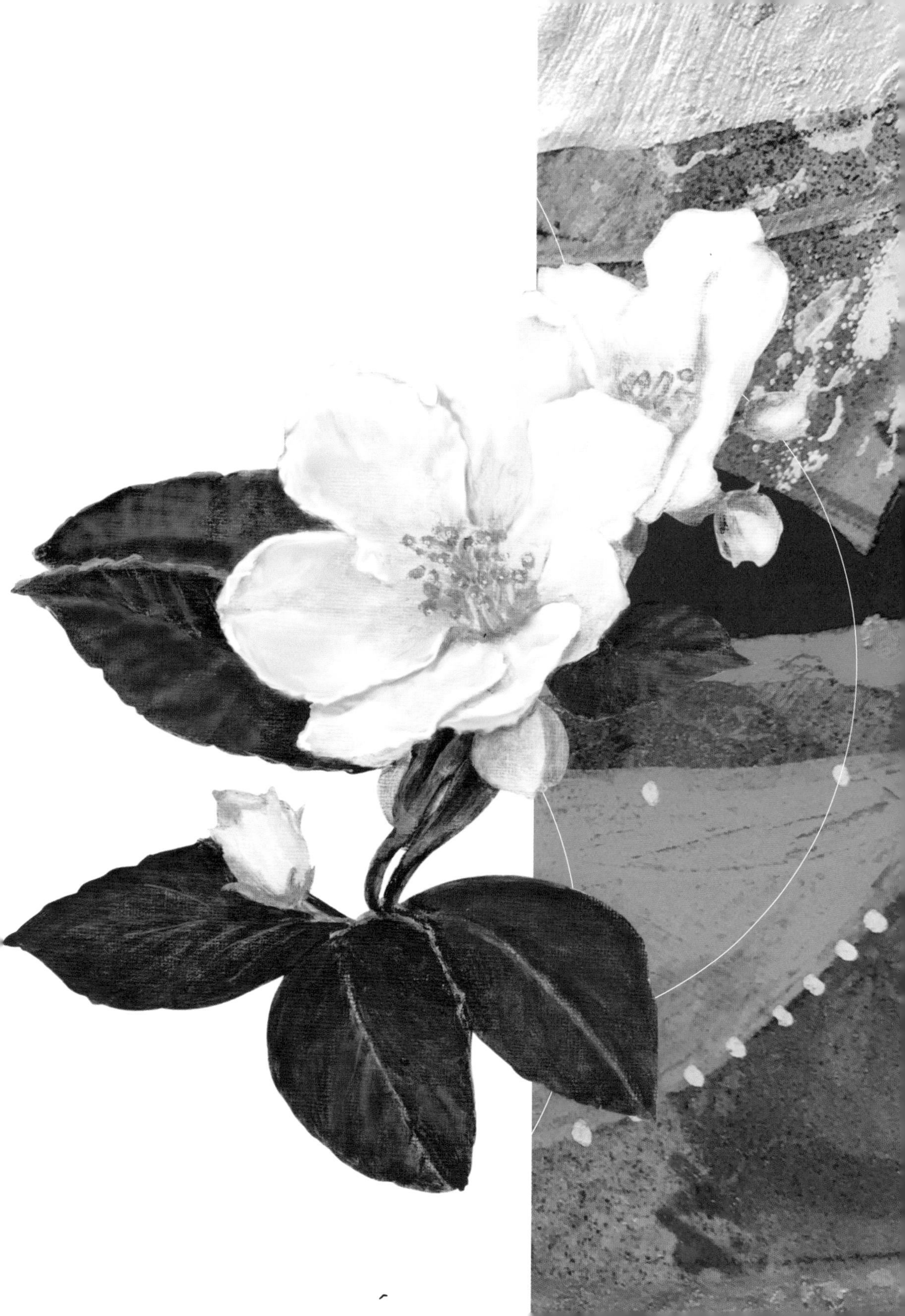

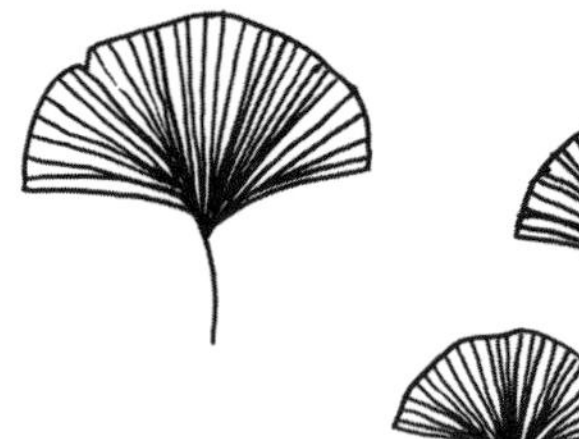

Love Lies Bleeding

LOVE LIES BLEEDING FLOWER ESSENCE WILL ASSIST YOU WITH:

- Releasing isolating patterns
- Uplifting and transcending consciousness
- Building compassionate understanding

Invocation

Take a trip into town or to a busy environment and take this flower essence with you. After consuming it, meditate and observe people around you. Notice within you what feelings arise. Can you see their suffering? What does humanity really need at this time? Reflect on this. Give yourself this gift of compassion first and foremost. Be ready for a transformation of the soul.

Also known as Pendant Amaranth or Velvet Flower, this annual flowering plant is an edible flower with many uses that can grow up to 8 feet (2.4 m) high. Love Lies Bleeding flower essence inspires Christ Consciousness, stirring deep compassion and feelings of empathy about the nature of suffering. If you have been isolating yourself or wrapping yourself in sadness lately, consider this potent healer. Love Lies Bleeding is about transcending that pain into understanding, from a deeply internal process to one that sees the suffering of all of humanity. Living in a place of compassion liberates the soul. This essence transforms feelings of alienation and isolation into feelings of connection with the matrix of the nature of human consciousness itself. You will understand that many souls are in pain also. You are not alone. This realization will bring you out of the small self into the whole self, where a more loving heart that is open to others begins to take root.

Pink Yarrow

PINK YARROW FLOWER ESSENCE WILL ASSIST YOU WITH:

- Bringing about emotional clarity
- Creating healthy boundaries for love
- Inspiring sovereignty of your energy

Invocation

Take this flower essence and then find a quiet place to sit. Close your eyes and envision your heart. See how it radiates so strongly inside you with so much power and warmth. Its nature is love because it is love, in and of itself. Feel the freedom that this love alone can bring to sustain you.

A flowering plant that is native to temperate regions of the Northern Hemisphere in Asia, Europe, and North America, Yarrow has a long history of human usage, including in Native American and Chinese divination rituals. The pink variety, however, seems to be native to California, and its flower essence is helpful for setting heart-based boundaries. Pink Yarrow establishes a clear energetic vibration inside oneself, replacing patterns of merging with others' emotions or frequently becoming oversympathetic that can cause the heart to lose some vital energy. Empaths, healers, therapists, and other guides may find this flower essence helpful for creating such boundaries. If you find yourself unable to distinguish your emotions from what others may be feeling, then Pink Yarrow could benefit you. It helps strengthen and inspire objectivity, creating space for more compassion without becoming enabling. You can use it to go from absorbing others' energy to radiating out love and understanding.

Rose

ROSE FLOWER ESSENCE WILL ASSIST YOU WITH:

- Motivating self-care practices
- Inspiring profound healing for the heart
- Sparking feelings of unconditional love

Invocation

Draw a warm bath, light candles, and place some rose flower petals in the bathwater. Take this flower essence and add a few drops to your bath. Notice your heart; how is it feeling? Continue to pay attention throughout your bath. Allow your heart to feel held and full. Give it the love and care it needs daily with the support of this essence.

A part of the vast genus *Rosa*, this woody perennial has more than 300 species, most native to Asia. The rose has a long worldwide history and is symbolic of the majesty of romance and divine love. Rose flower essence is a true healer for the heart chakra. It inspires feelings of forgiveness and unconditional love for oneself along with a clearer connection to the divine. It helps you prioritize self-care, especially related to matters of the heart. It strengthens and emboldens the heart's knowledge and wisdom so you can lead your life from a place of the power of love within. Rose also aids in mending and nurturing the heart from past disappointments. It cools the loving nature and allows forgiveness to flow with grace. Warmth and radiance emerge from the heart, providing courage, strength, and grounding in the divine mystery.

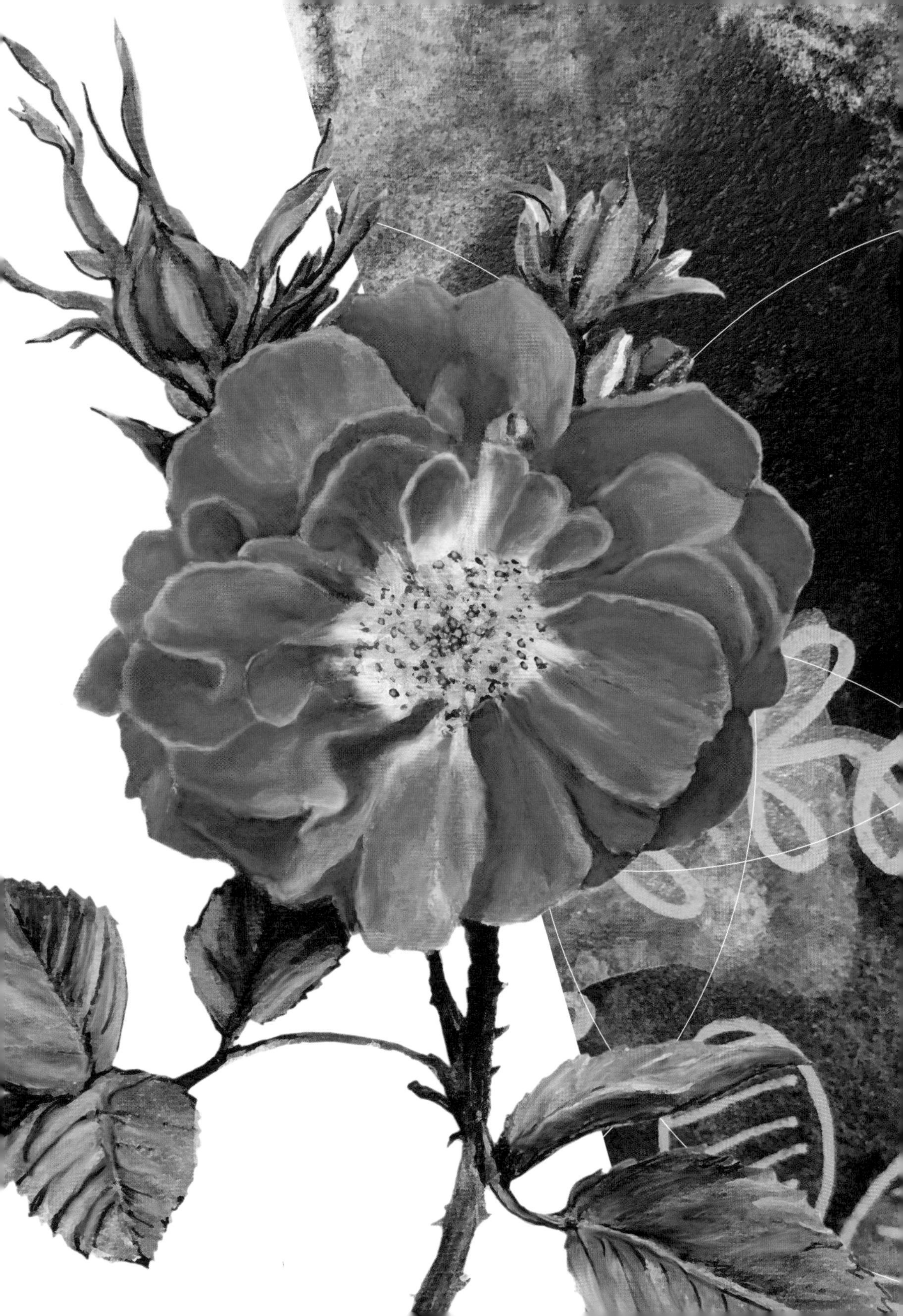

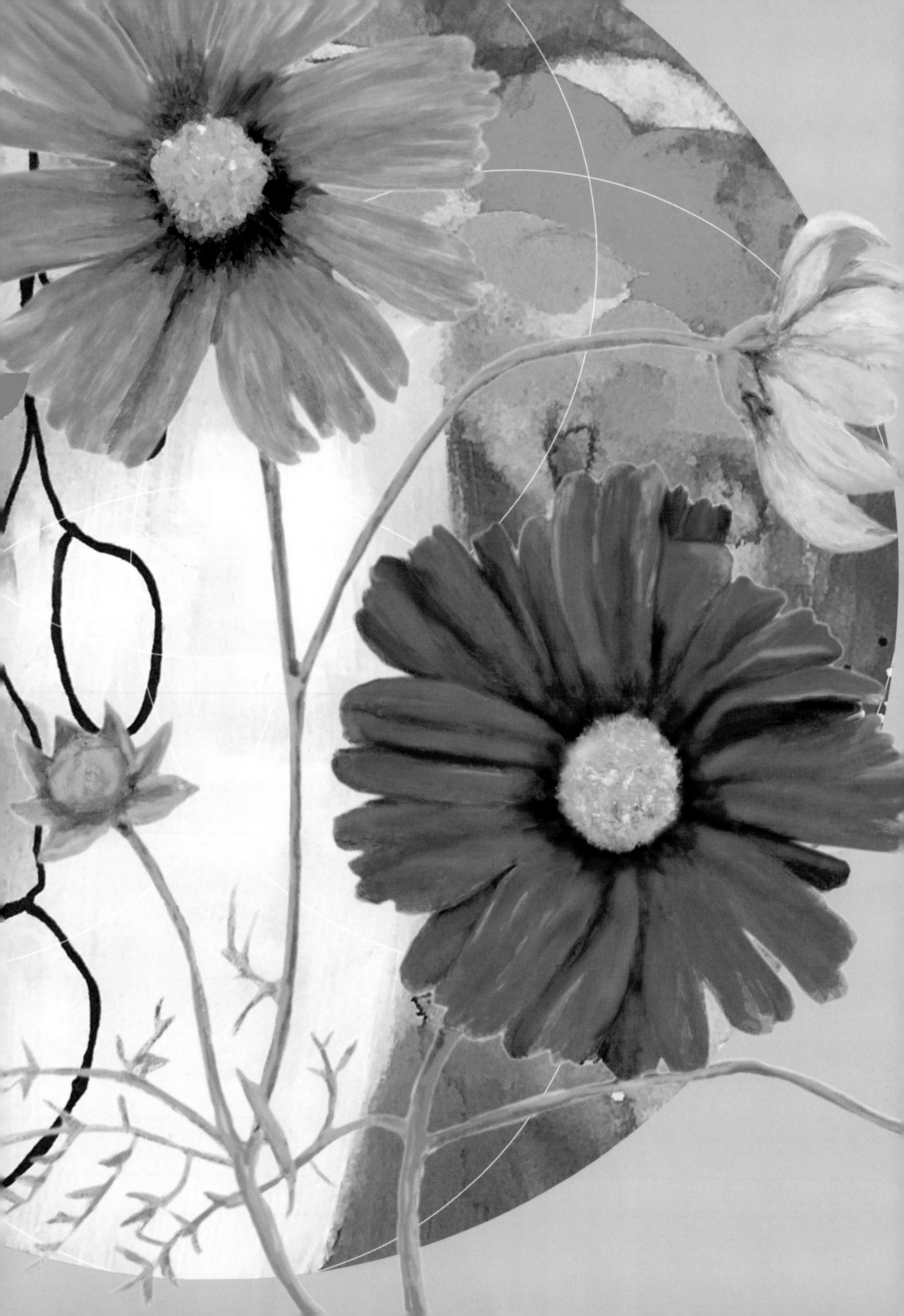

7 Flower Essences for Clairvoyance

"

Practice listening to your intuition, your inner voice; ask questions; be curious; see what you see; hear what you hear; and then act upon what you know to be true. These intuitive powers were given to your soul at birth.

— Clarissa Pinkola Estés

I believe we all are psychic. We're all intuitive, and we have gut instincts that we can sense or feel. Our senses have an innate wisdom that goes beyond the rational mind. The more we can quiet our analytical mind and discover silence and our inner voice, the more truth we can uncover inside ourselves. Our intuitive self always has our best interest at heart. It is a quiet whisper or gentle voice that desires to guide us to the truth that our heart can understand and feel. Learning to trust the intuitive self is a practice. But the more we understand that wisdom already lies inside of us, the more we can trust ourselves to lead the way. This is the beginning of a journey into a life that is truthful and aligned. The flower essences in this chapter can help open up and enhance your intuitive capabilities. Trust the guidance that comes from within and enjoy the journey of listening to your heart's guidance.

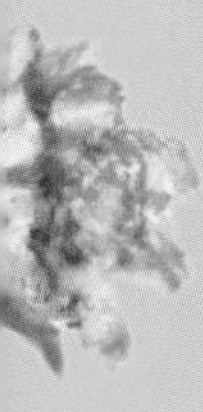

Angel's Trumpet

ANGEL'S TRUMPET FLOWER ESSENCE WILL ASSIST YOU WITH:

- Opening up the channels to higher states
- Letting go of the fear of death
- Rebirthing the soul into new states of consciousness

Invocation

Take your Angel's Trumpet essence with you during times of major transition or major life occurrences. If you are saying goodbye to someone you love, this essence can be of an energetic comfort to you or your loved one, if they are willing. Just having it nearby can be a blessing. Angel's Trumpet is wonderful for other times of rebirthing or spiritual surrender. Use it with care and reverence.

Growing up to 26 feet (7.9 m) tall, this tree-like shrub produces numerous hanging, fragrant flowers and is native to Ecuador and Columbia. It has a rich history of use in Shamanism for healing and divination. It is best known for its ability to help a soul surrender to death, especially if there is fear or resistance. Angel's Trumpet assists the soul in its own liberation and allows for consciousness to take deeper root. The gift of clairvoyance and guidance for tapping into other realms can also take place. Use Angel's Trumpet for Shamanic rituals or other rebirth experiences in which the soul can experience profound opening and transformation. Whenever a loved one is leaving their body, this essence can be there for potent and loving support.

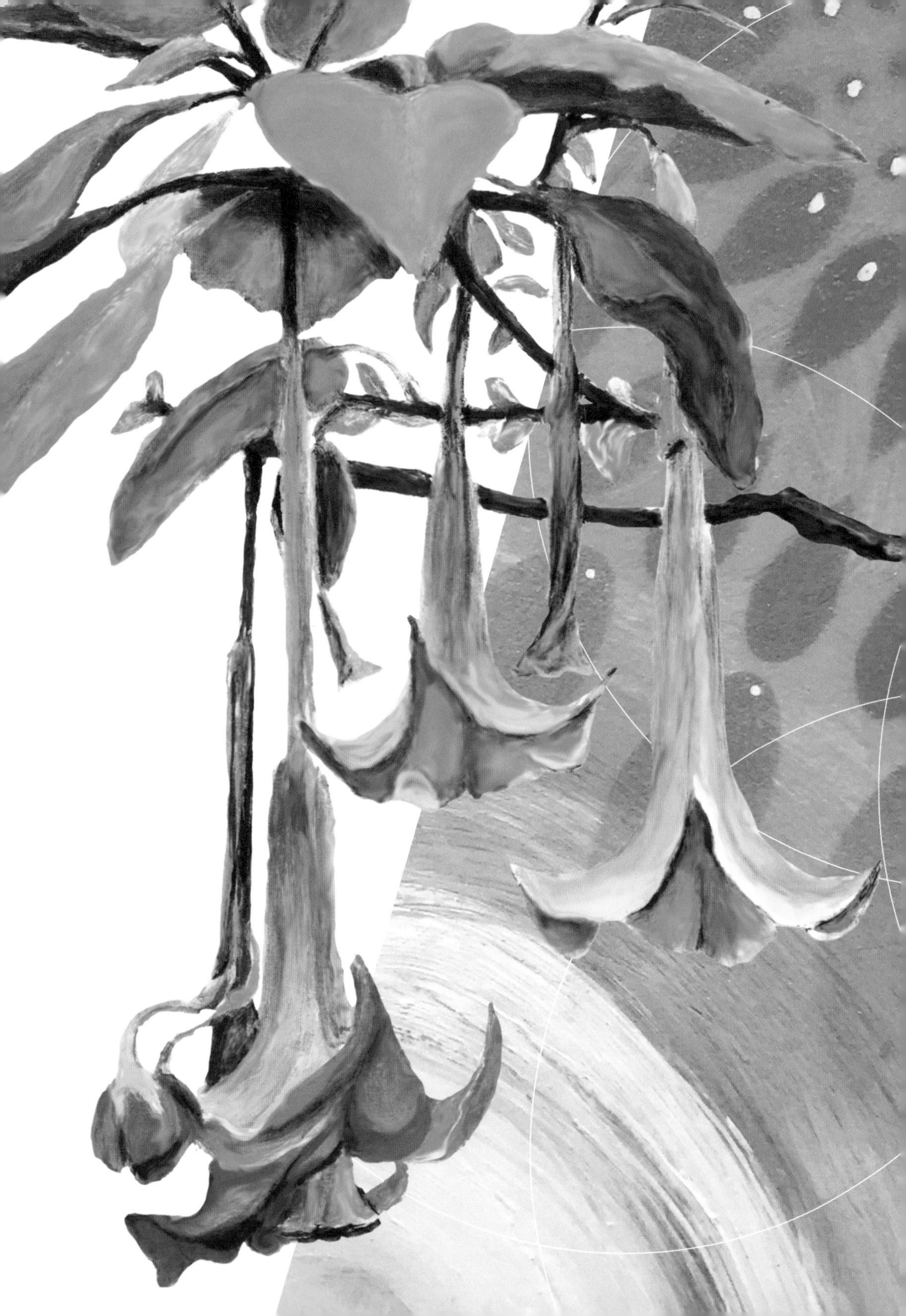

Angelica

ANGELICA FLOWER ESSENCE WILL ASSIST YOU WITH:

- Feeling angelic protection
- Healing issues of spiritual abandonment
- Support in times of birth, death, and other major life occurrences

Invocation

Hold this flower essence softly against your chest and say a prayer to the angelic realm. Ask that you may have more angelic presence in your life. Ask for protection, guidance, or whatever comes to you. Take Angelica knowing that your angels are closer to you now.

Also called Wild Celery or Garden Angelica, this biennial flower, known for its healing properties and edible components, can grow to be more than 8 feet (2.4 m) tall and is native to Europe and Asia. At various times in life, we can feel disconnected from source or a higher power, and often we begin to overanalyze and intellectualize matters. In these times, our rational mind has become too loud and we have lost sight of our intuition. Taking Angelica can help restore the balance and help us feel spiritual presence and guidance from higher powers. By taking this essence, you may feel more connected to the angelic realm and to angelic protection and guidance. This allows for deeper integration of our true nature to take place—one that is grounded in both the physical world and the cosmic afterlife.

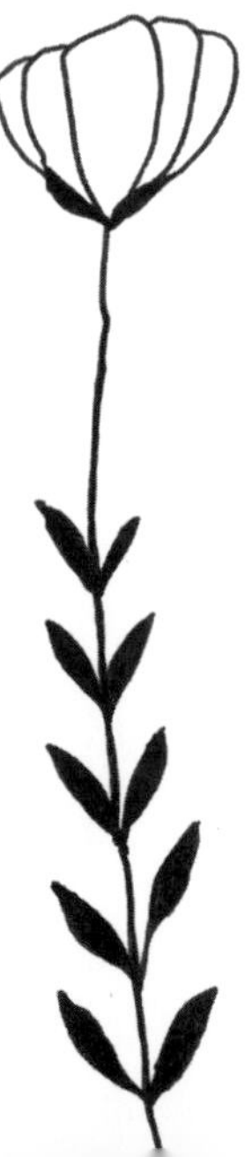

Aspen

ASPEN FLOWER ESSENCE WILL ASSIST YOU WITH:

- Healing fears of what is not known
- Restoring trust
- Balancing an overly intuitive or sensitive soul

Invocation

Find a quiet spot to sit in nature and take your Aspen flower essence with you. Lay out a blanket, sit or lie down on it, and breathe deeply into your lower body and feet, asking the earth to ground you as you take this essence. Aspen flower essence assists in balancing psychic downloads for overly sensitive souls so the messages they receive are not so frequent and debilitating.

Native to the temperate regions of Asia, Europe, and various other parts of the world, this deciduous tree can grow up to 130 feet (39.6 m) tall. Aspen flower essence helps highly sensitive souls balance the number of psychic downloads they receive. If the upper chakras open up too widely in relationship to the physical body, you can feel too readily like you are floating or under psychic attack. Sometimes these feelings can produce intense fears and paranoia. This flower essence helps restore balance and trust when using intuition and when determining what is based in fear or past trauma versus what is inner knowing. Harmony among all the energy centers and the emotional, spiritual, and mental bodies can then take place. Use Aspen when your clairvoyance feels out of tune and apprehensive.

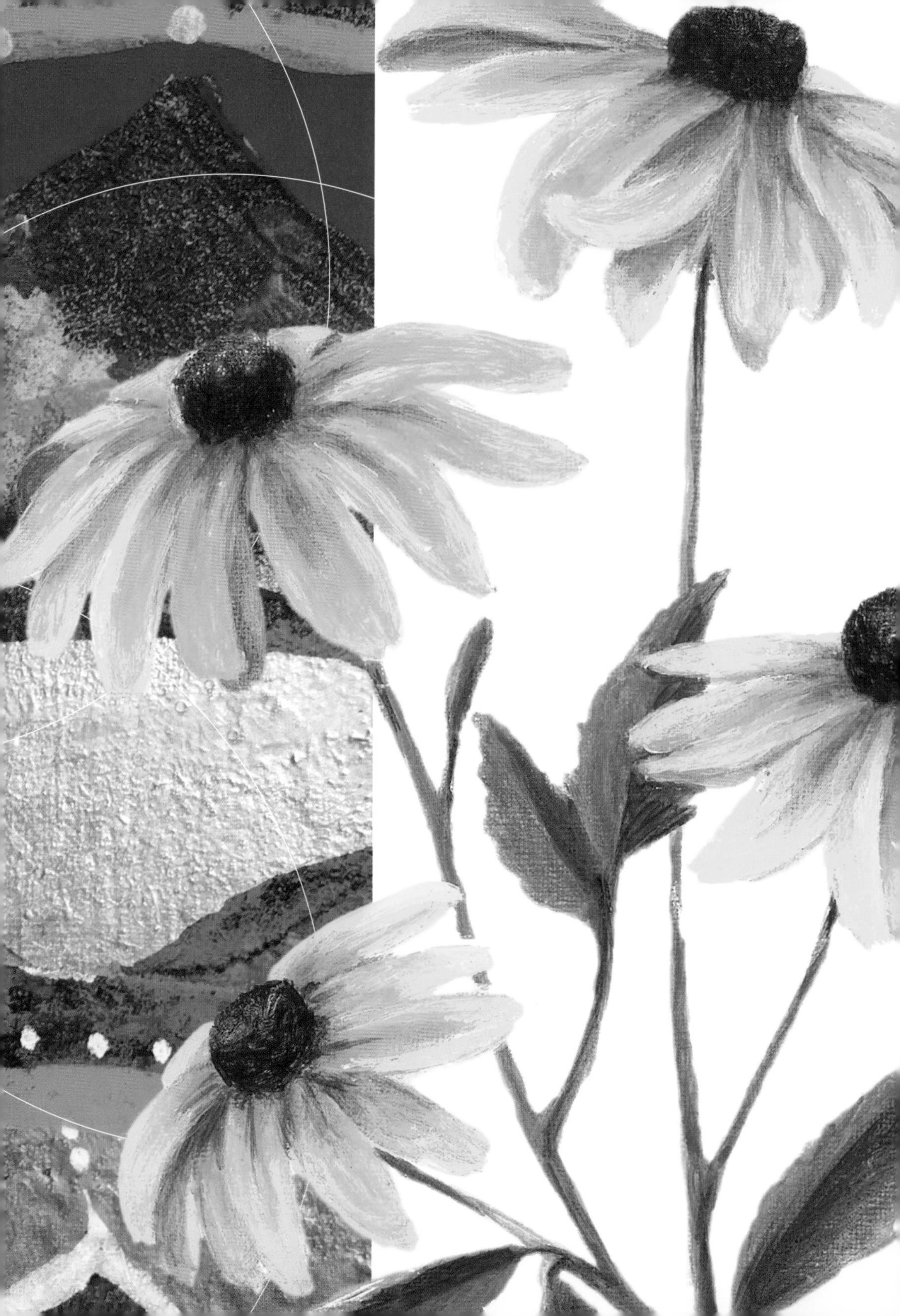

Black-Eyed Susan

BLACK-EYED SUSAN FLOWER ESSENCE WILL ASSIST YOU WITH:

- Integrating the shadow self
- Awakening insight and awareness
- Transforming all parts of the psyche

Invocation

Take this flower essence with you the next time you visit a therapist, bodyworker, or healer. Take Black-Eyed Susan right before your session and share your intention to integrate all parts of yourself, including repressed events that may still be affecting your present-day awareness. Allow whatever comes up to be an important part of your transformation. Hold yourself gently in this new awareness.

Part of the sunflower family, this North American plant grows readily in almost all the states as well as in parts of China. Its glorious yellow leaves and dark brown center make it noticeable in gardens and in the wild. Black-Eyed Susan flower essence helps awaken all parts of the self for integration and clearer insight. When the shadow side of our self has been repressed, we can act out in unconscious ways, not knowing where the emotional reaction is coming from. This essence can bring the subconscious to light so that we may act instead from integrity and self-awareness. Take this essence if you feel you are repressing past trauma and you notice patterns in your life that have caused harm to you and others. This powerful healer will help bring together all parts of the self so you can awaken to truth with clearer insight and knowing.

Cerato

CERATO FLOWER ESSENCE WILL ASSIST YOU WITH:

- Trusting your intuition
- Building self-reliance
- Cultivating sovereignty

Invocation

Take this flower essence before you begin to freewrite in your journal. Ask for the guidance of your higher or intuitive self. Then begin to write the things you know are true in your life. Allow your hand to write continuously and the words to flow without effort. Be amazed and trust in your inner knowing.

Native to Tibet and parts of China, this flowering shrub has pale blue blooms that turn to autumnal colors as the seasons change. Cerato assists us in trusting our intuition, our inner guidance, and ourselves. It alleviates the need to constantly seek others' opinions and advice, which can cause confusion and overthinking. This essence helps relieve self-doubt and uncertainty and bring in sovereignty and decision-making confidence. The gift of Cerato flower essence is that of trusting your own inner wisdom and knowledge so that you can move through life with confidence and ease.

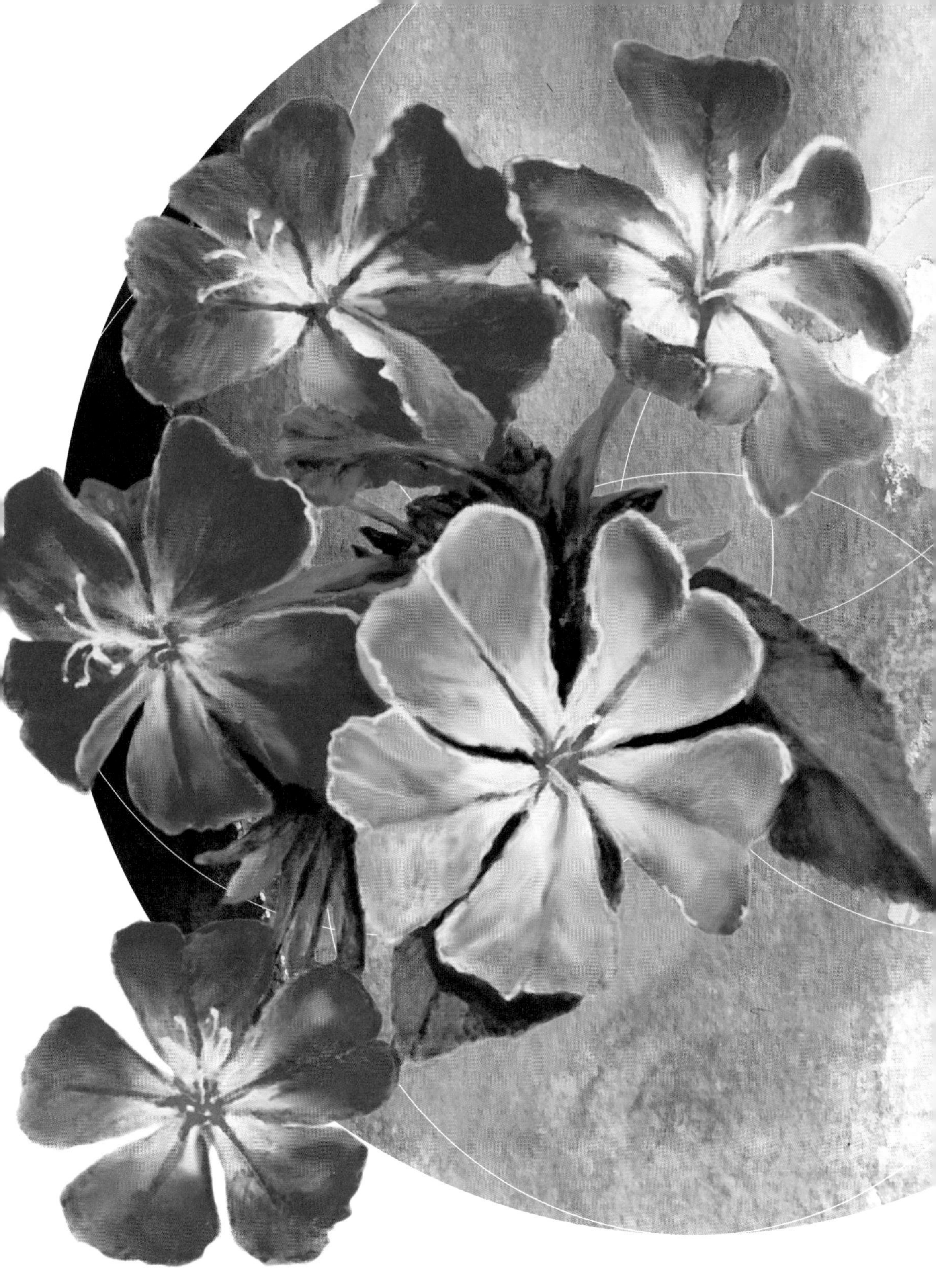

Cosmos

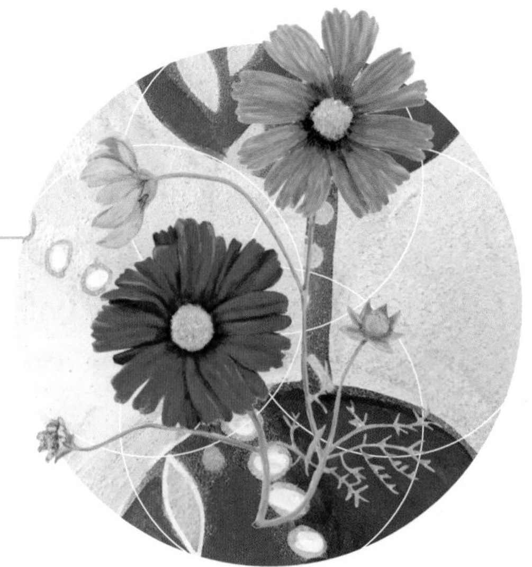

COSMOS FLOWER ESSENCE WILL ASSIST YOU WITH:

- Expressing yourself clearly
- Finding coherence between ideas and speech
- Focusing when overwhelmed by too many ideas

Invocation

Take this flower essence before beginning a speech or going to a gathering. Say the mantra "I express my ideas with flow and grace" three times or until you feel confident. Trust that you can express yourself with clarity.

An ornamental plant native to the Americas, Cosmos has beautiful reddish-purple petals with a yellow center. When the nervous system becomes overreactive (which is common in our overstimulated modern world), the coherence of our thoughts and speech can become overexcited or confusing. Frustration and annoyance can set in when we can't quite express what we are feeling or trying to convey. Enter the beloved Cosmos flower essence, which helps bring about clarity in thought and word. Disorganized speech becomes fluid and orderly, and we are able to tap into intuition to express inspired ideas and insights. Take this essence whenever you are feeling overwhelmed by the world and notice your ability to express yourself becoming disoriented. Let your true disposition come forth with ease in your verbal expression.

Monkshood

MONKSHOOD FLOWER ESSENCE WILL ASSIST YOU WITH:

- Inspiring spiritual leadership
- Cultivating courage
- Activating powerful clairvoyance

Invocation

The next time you sit down to meditate and tune in to your intuition, take this flower essence. Allow Monkshood to open up your psychic channels so that you may fully receive this blessing. Allow it to seep deep into your cells, knowing you are held in this new ability.

A flowering plant from the buttercup family, this wildflower is native to North America, where it often grows in moist areas of the forest. Monkshood flower essence assists in the integration of our expanded intuitive and psychic abilities. Oftentimes these psychic gifts can be shut down due to past trauma or fear of what may arise. This flower essence helps bring union and balance to those centers. It also helps us cultivate the courage to understand our inner guidance and therefore show up in life as a leader who follows the wisdom of the heart. The gift of Monkshood is integration of kind and moral values that can transform you into a true teacher or guide.

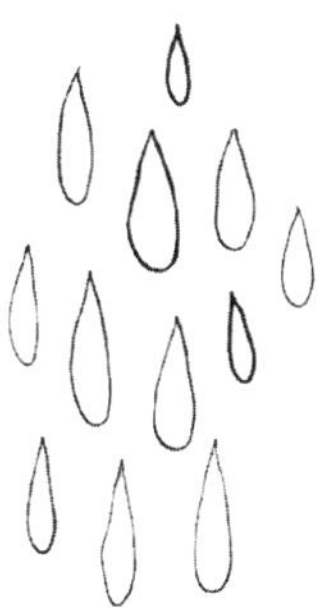

Queen Anne's Lace

QUEEN ANNE'S LACE FLOWER ESSENCE WILL ASSIST YOU WITH:

- Clearing up projections or emotional debris
- Integrating intuition and psychic abilities
- Harmonizing the lower and higher chakras

Invocation

Take this essence to a field of wildflowers, or just sit under a tree. After taking it, look up at the sky, then feel the support of the ground below you. Close your eyes and notice how you are held by both earth and sky. Allow your intuition to open and show you where next to go in life.

Also known as Wild Carrot, this abundant wildflower is native to temperate parts of Europe and Asia. It is a biennial plant that has white, lacy petals clustered together. Queen Anne's Lace flower essence assists with healing emotional imbalances and projections. It bestows the gifts of wholly integrated clairvoyance, which allows you to see clearly, removing emotional debris from your psychic channels. The gift of this lacy flower is harmony of all chakras so that our spiritual insight and clairvoyant abilities are grounded and true. It can help stabilize energies, meaning you can stay connected to the earth while receiving guidance from the higher realms. Enjoy the gift of this essence, much needed in our times, and allow it to show you the path of harmony.

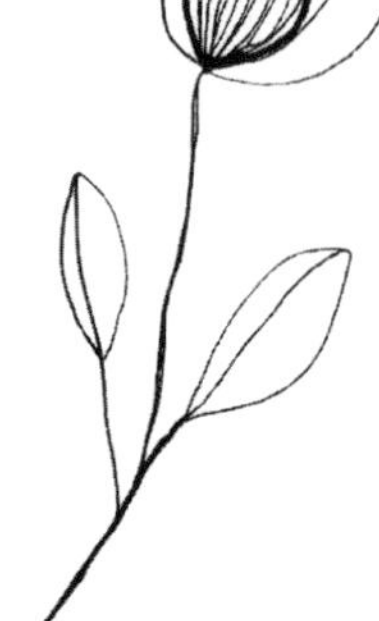

Star Tulip

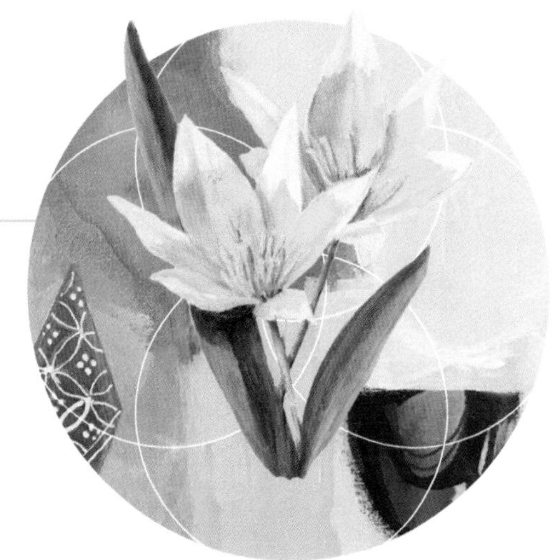

STAR TULIP FLOWER ESSENCE WILL ASSIST YOU WITH:

- Meditating and turning within
- Softening to more receptivity
- Tuning in to intuition and the dreamworld

Invocation

Before bedtime, light some candles and take Star Tulip flower essence. Begin to breathe into your heart along with your upper chakras or centers. Follow your inhalations and exhalations for as long as you can, until you become sleepy. Allow the dreamworld to show you revelations and guidance from your higher self.

Also known at Cat's Ears and native to the United States, this perennial herb is part of the lily family and has hairy petals with narrow sepals in the center. Star Tulip flower essence assists in the expansion and flowering of the heart. It helps the soul listen to higher guidance and intuition, thus becoming more aware of subtle energies. This essence can help the divine feminine part of ourselves, the part that allows for sensitivity and receptivity, to be a larger part of daily life. Prayer, meditation, and tuning in to the dreamworld all become more activated. Allow Star Tulip to bestow its dreamy gifts onto your soul with grace.

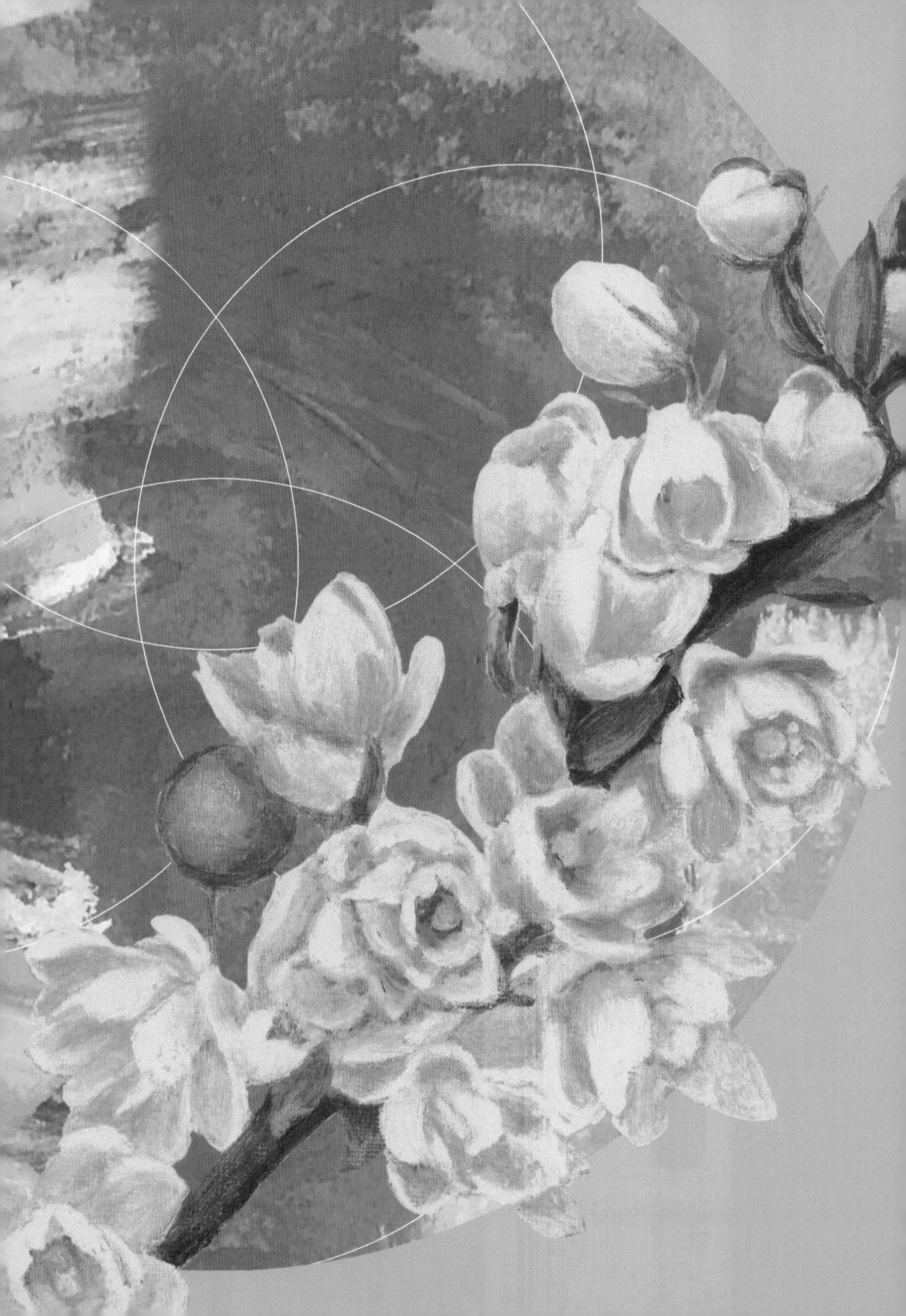

8 Flower Essences for Courage

"

Courage is the most important of all the virtues because without courage, you can't practice any other virtue consistently.

—Maya Angelou

The root word for courage is *cor*, a Latin word that means "heart." According to Brené Brown, the word in its earliest form meant "to speak one's mind by telling all one's heart." It is essential to live life courageously through the heart. How can we receive what we desire unless we go after it fearlessly and unapologetically? Courage keeps the heart aflame and thus rewarded—a virtue of utmost value that spreads into every aspect of life. Let's dive into the floral realms to understand which essences can help us show up bravely and allow ourselves to be seen.

Larch

LARCH FLOWER ESSENCE WILL ASSIST YOU WITH:

- Self-assurance
- Spontaneous action
- Expansive creativity

Invocation

Take this flower essence when you want to build courage and free up creative expression. Before you begin a new painting or start a performance or any other artistic endeavor, let Larch give you confidence and liberate your creative self.

Larch is an appropriate healer for courage, as it helps one overcome self-doubt and insecurity. Native to the mountainous regions of central Europe and readily found in England, this pinkish-red flower grows on the larch tree, which can live for up to 250 years. Larch allows us to release shame and lack of confidence, so we can view ourselves as fully capable of tasks. It alleviates fear of expression, allowing our true courageous and creative voice to come through. Thus, Larch can be helpful to artistically inclined people who often find themselves doubting their skills. Larch expands the soul from a limited state to one that expresses itself spontaneously and with bravery. This incredible essence frees up internal energy to become more creatively expressed and confident.

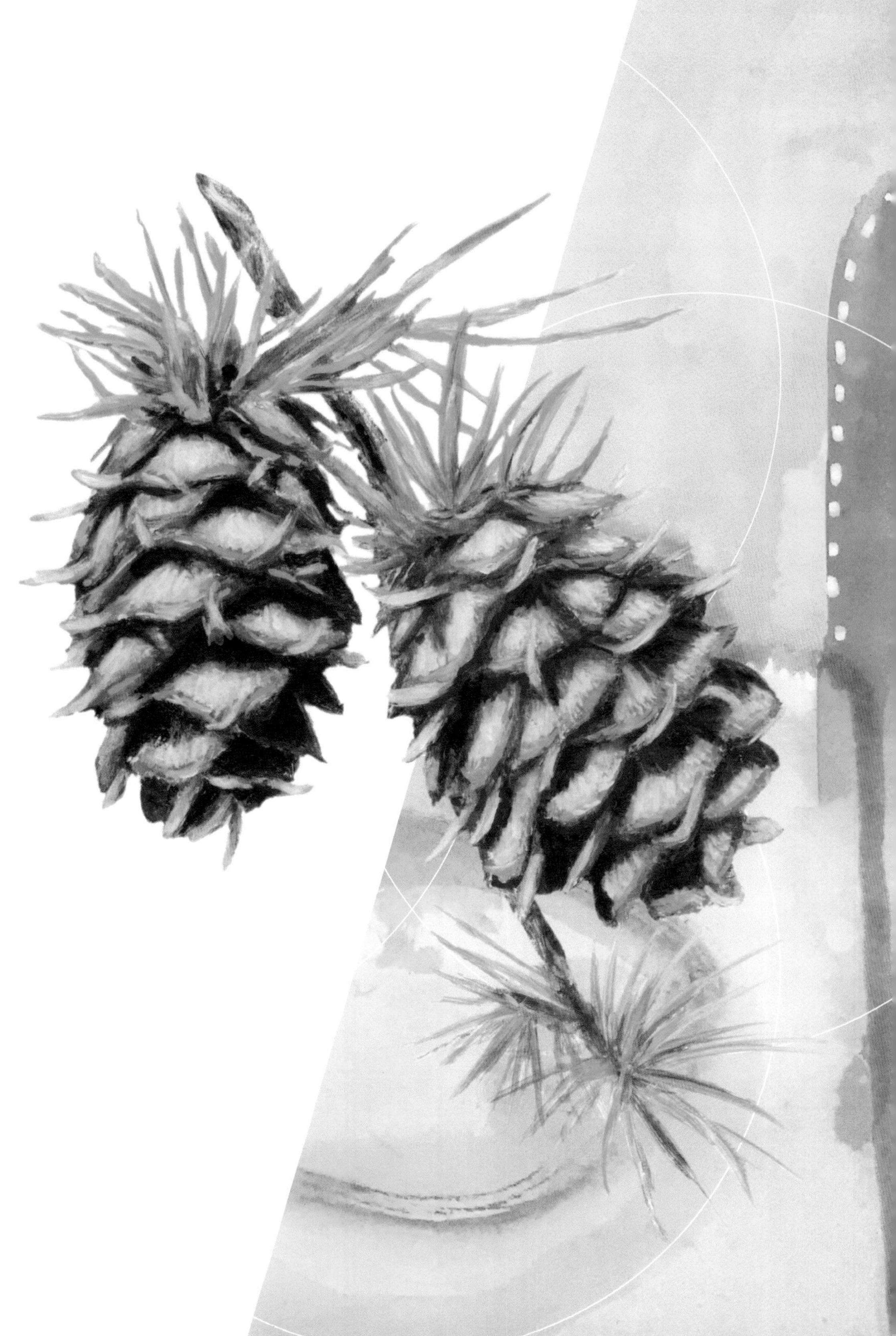

Gentian

GENTIAN FLOWER ESSENCE WILL ASSIST YOU WITH:

- Restoring confidence
- Building perseverance
- Establishing fortitude and unwavering trust

Invocation

After a setback, make some time for self-care and take this flower essence to build up encouragement. Gentian flower essence allows for the integration of all parts of the subconscious and an optimistic point of view when life gives us hurdles.

Gentiana, a genus species of flowering plants, is most often recognized as an intense deep-blue flower in the shape of a trumpet. However, in this case *Gentian* refers to a purple biennial plant that can be found in northern Europe. It blooms between July and September. Gentian helps with perseverance and optimism after a perceived setback. Taking this essence could benefit you when you're feeling discouraged and disenchanted after things go wrong. A Gentian remedy will help the soul become courageous and strong, with a resilience that is full of hope and a more positive outlook on life. Doubts will transform into embodiments of a deeper faith. The intention of this essence is to teach souls that after failure comes growth and learning, which leads to a clearer understanding of one's own life journey.

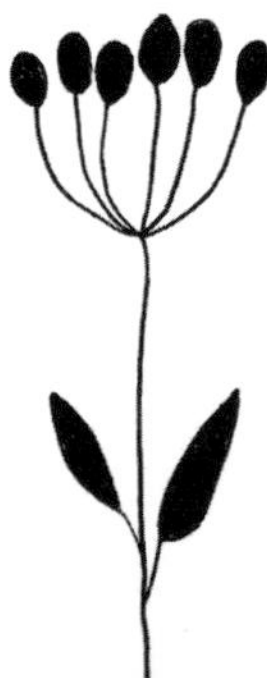

Mountain Pride

MOUNTAIN PRIDE FLOWER ESSENCE WILL ASSIST YOU WITH:

- Building assertiveness
- Having the courage to take a stand
- Taking action in the world for the greater good

Invocation

Before going on a hike or an outdoor adventure, take this flower essence to embody warrior-like qualities. Mountain Pride flower essence is good for brave acts of compassion in this world. It gets us in touch with our inner masculine nature and builds the strength we need to go out and get things done.

Native to California, Mountain Pride is a magenta perennial flower that blooms from June to August. Its flower essence helps us find our true purpose in life. It also brings about a direct, warrior-like spirituality that can see things head-on and transform them. Mountain Pride promotes healing for a withdrawn, dissatisfied, and passive attitude. It helps turn lack of confidence into the empowerment needed to stand up for what's right. Take this flower essence if you wish to move forward in life with strength, fortitude, and goodness in your heart. Mountain Pride is a gift if you wish to learn to speak up and take positive action in this world with bravery and truth on your side.

Oregon Grape

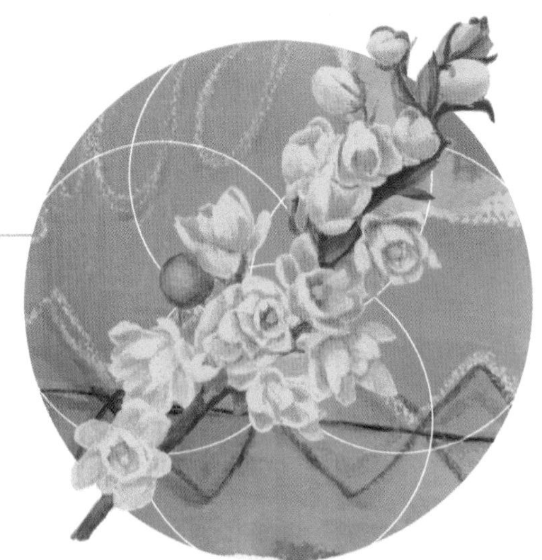

OREGON GRAPE FLOWER ESSENCE WILL ASSIST YOU WITH:

- Trusting others
- Having a positive outlook about the world
- Feeling warmth toward humanity

Invocation

Reflect and write about why you mistrust people so much. Then take this flower essence to help with your cynicism about humanity. When you want to inspire and connect with others, allow Oregon Grape flower essence to build the courage you need to let others into your world.

Native to the North Pacific coastal region, from southern British Columbia to central Oregon, Oregon Grape is commonly found in Douglas fir forests. Its yellow flowers turn into bluish-purple berries, which are used medicinally. Oregon Grape flower essence releases paranoia about what others think of you and restores courage and faith. It enhances your ability to believe in your own power as a sovereign soul who can trust humankind. In this way, Oregon Grape is helpful for courage: One cannot begin to trust without being vulnerable enough to act and think in brave new ways. Viewing others as dangerous and untrustworthy keeps a protective shield over the heart, but Oregon Grape reveals a more positive outlook and a courageous heart that can come shining forth.

Penstemon

PENSTEMON FLOWER ESSENCE WILL ASSIST YOU WITH:

- Persevering during hard times
- Building up inner fortitude
- Allowing for deep transformation

Invocation

When you need to face the world during a stressful time, take this flower essence first thing in the morning to build up courage. Say some positive affirmations out loud, if you wish. The day is yours to seize. Penstemon flower essence helps us tap into reservoirs of resilience and bravery.

Native to the West Coast of the United States, this low-forming perennial has tubular blue-lavender buds. Penstemon provides great strength, courage, and perseverance during challenging life circumstances. If you are feeling sorry for yourself, you may benefit from taking this flower essence. Those who have been through unusually hard circumstances may feel more ease and grace after taking Penstemon. Those circumstances could include the loss of something special, which causes a soul to lose faith and feel pity or intense despair. Penstemon brings about more courageous energy for that soul, rebuilding it with feelings of trust and hope. Take Penstemon if you feel unable to confront harsh circumstances and desire a braver and more faithful outlook on life.

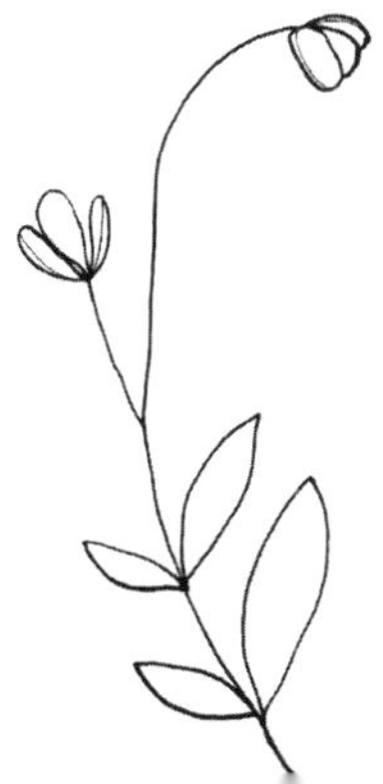

Pink Monkeyflower

PINK MONKEYFLOWER FLOWER ESSENCE WILL ASSIST YOU WITH:

- Being vulnerable enough to share your truth
- Opening the heart
- Taking an emotional risk

Invocation

Before having a heart-to-heart talk with someone with whom you feel called to share vulnerable feelings, take this flower essence to give you courage. Pink Monkeyflower essence is all about opening the heart when feeling emotionally vulnerable. Breathe in deeply and know that this is how you transform your life and relationships.

Part of the *Mimulus* genus, which includes more than 150 species in a variety of colors, these flowers are identified by their mouth-like shape. The Pink Monkeyflower, which grows in riparian habitats, inspires courage by allowing us to take emotional risks that bring about openness and authenticity. This essence heals feelings of rejection, shame, and unworthiness—all emotions that are toxic to one's liberation. Pink Monkeyflower further assists in healing deep fears of being seen in one's most vulnerable state. Souls who would benefit from this essence are more than just shy; they are covering up trauma or childhood wounds. This essence can help those who are highly sensitive and carry a deep sense of shame and unworthiness. Pink Monkeyflower works to heal such emotional pain and bring forth courage for sharing truthfully.

Red Clover

RED CLOVER FLOWER ESSENCE WILL ASSIST YOU WITH:

- Embodying a calm presence
- Becoming more self-aware
- Feeling grounded in courage

Invocation

Take this flower essence while sitting under a strong tree and breathing slowly and deeply into your core. Red Clover flower essence assists you in grounded bravery so you can face stressful situations with ease.

Red Clover, an edible flowering perennial with reddish-pink buds, is native to northwest Africa, Europe, and western Asia. These tiny buds are used medicinally in the herbal world. And Red Clover flower essence's energetic healing properties are perfect for working with courage. Red Clover provides us with a calm, grounded presence when we are faced with adversity. In the midst of chaos, this essence allows us to feel brave and centered. People who become easily anxious in groups, losing their identity and their confidence, can benefit from taking Red Clover. This powerful bud balances out the energy so you can move forward in life with self-awareness and with a brave and calm presence.

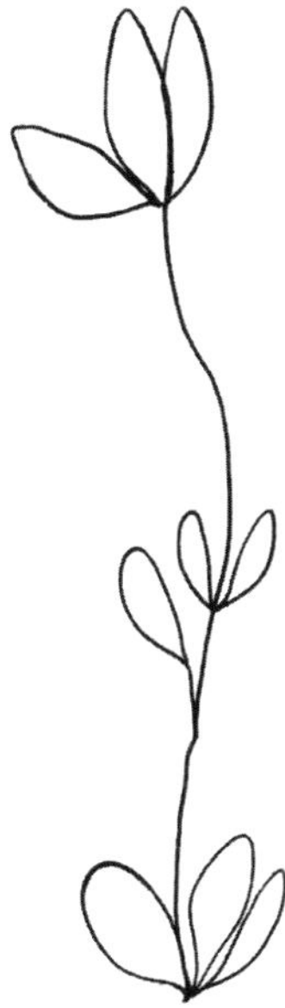

Rock Rose

ROCK ROSE FLOWER ESSENCE WILL ASSIST YOU WITH:

- Building strength when facing intense challenges
- Transcending fear into courage
- Feeling support during a crisis

Invocation

Use Rock Rose when you are faced with a traumatic event and need to call upon your inner courage to see you through. Sit in the sunlight, breathe deeply, and take this flower essence, knowing that this too shall pass. Allow Rock Rose to warm your spirit with strength.

A yellow, saucer-like flower native to most of Europe, Rock Rose is a trailing evergreen plant that blooms from May to July. Although it blooms for just a short time, it produces a plethora of flowers in arid, sunny spots. This powerful flower essence calls upon deep courage for our souls when we're in the middle of a crisis or an extreme challenge. When traumatic events cause pain or fear of death, this flower essence is the one to call upon. Rock Rose inspires warmth and sunlight in the human heart so that it can show up to intense challenges with transcendent bravery. This essence also is appropriate when faced with the ego's fear of death. Use Rock Rose whenever immense strength and courage are called upon during life's most challenging occurrences.

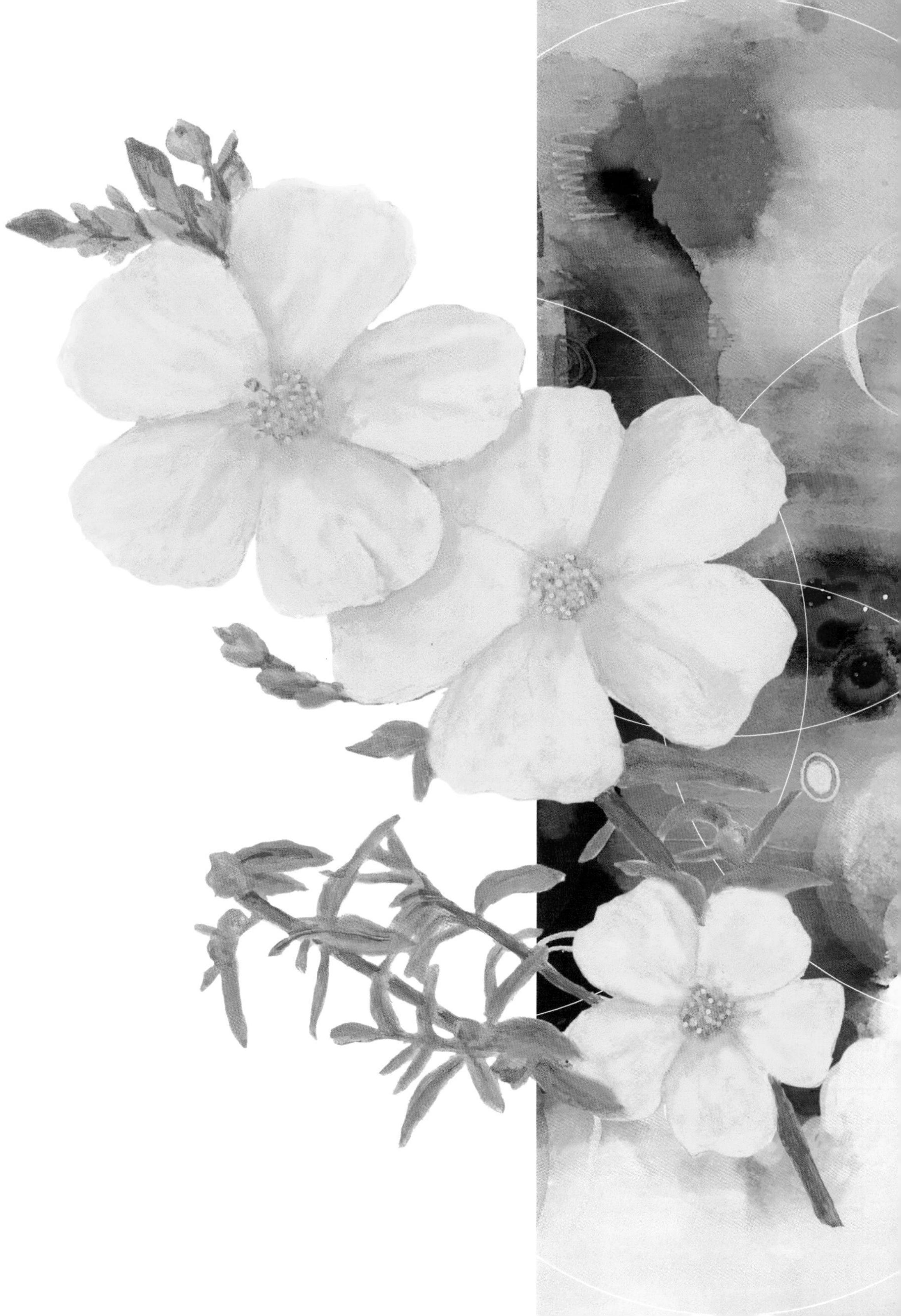

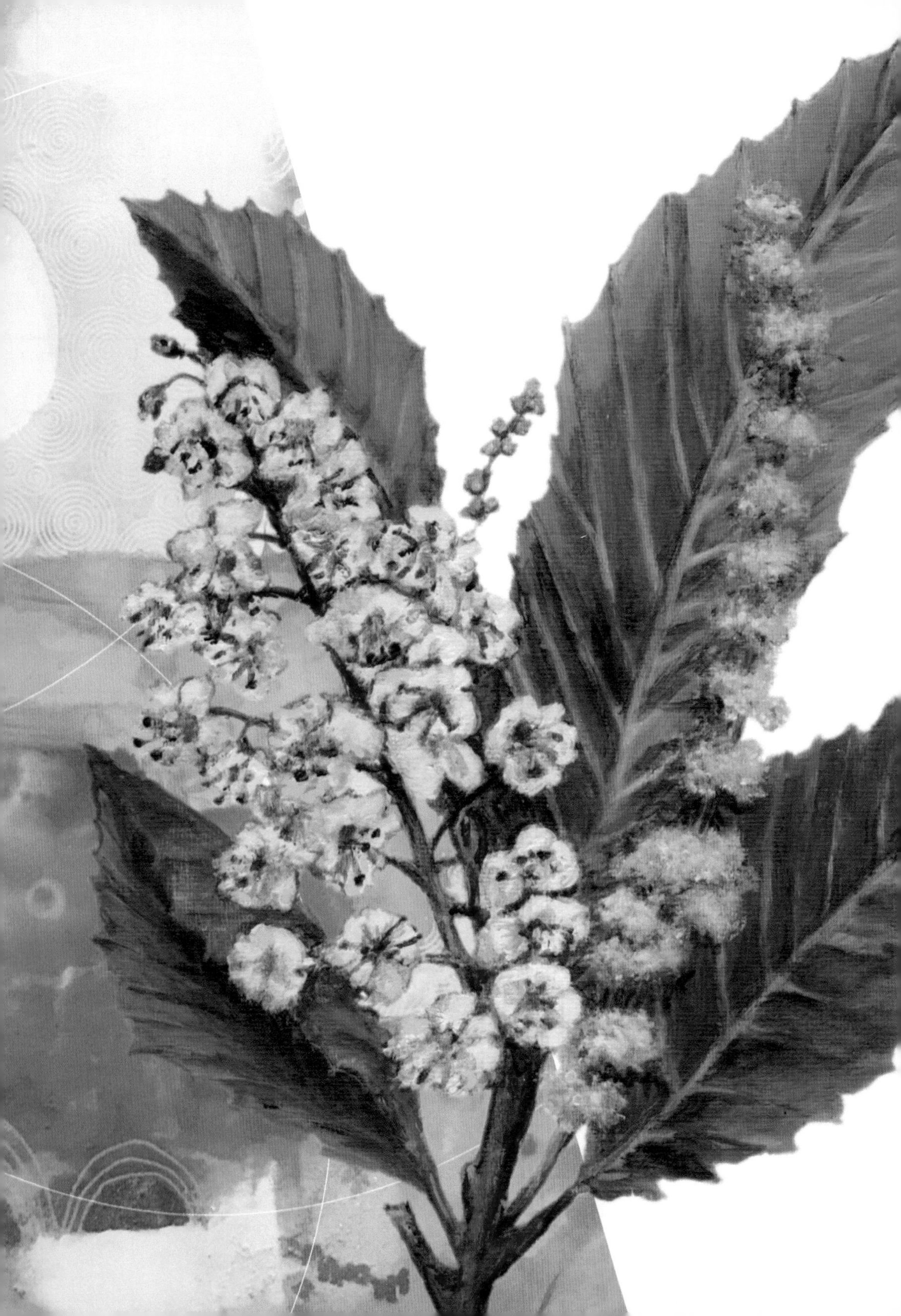

Sweet Chestnut

SWEET CHESTNUT FLOWER ESSENCE WILL ASSIST YOU WITH:

- Lifting up out of despair
- Experiencing rebirth and transformation
- Finding the courage to trust again

Invocation

Wrap yourself up in a blanket, light a candle, and take this flower essence when facing deep despair. Allow Sweet Chestnut to uplift your spirit gently and give you an opportunity for profound spiritual transformation.

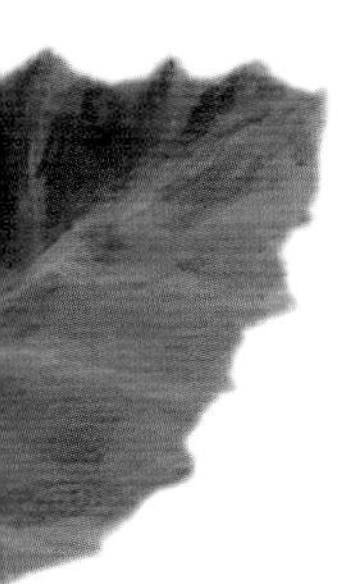

Native to southern Europe, parts of Asia Minor, and throughout temperate climates, this deciduous tree produces a flowering plant that has been used in cooking for thousands of years. Sweet Chestnut is an immensely healing plant used when courage and faith are needed the most. When you are in deep anguish or sorrow and experiencing intense darkness, this essence helps lift you out of such acute pain and despair. It also is appropriate for those feeling isolated and alone in their pain. Sweet Chestnut assists in giving the soul bravery to lift out of extreme mental, emotional, or physical states. This essence is all about the power of transformation and the knowledge that rebirth of the spirit is possible. It can help you move from pain to more expansive and aware states of consciousness. By taking Sweet Chestnut, you can be brave enough to feel some faith again.

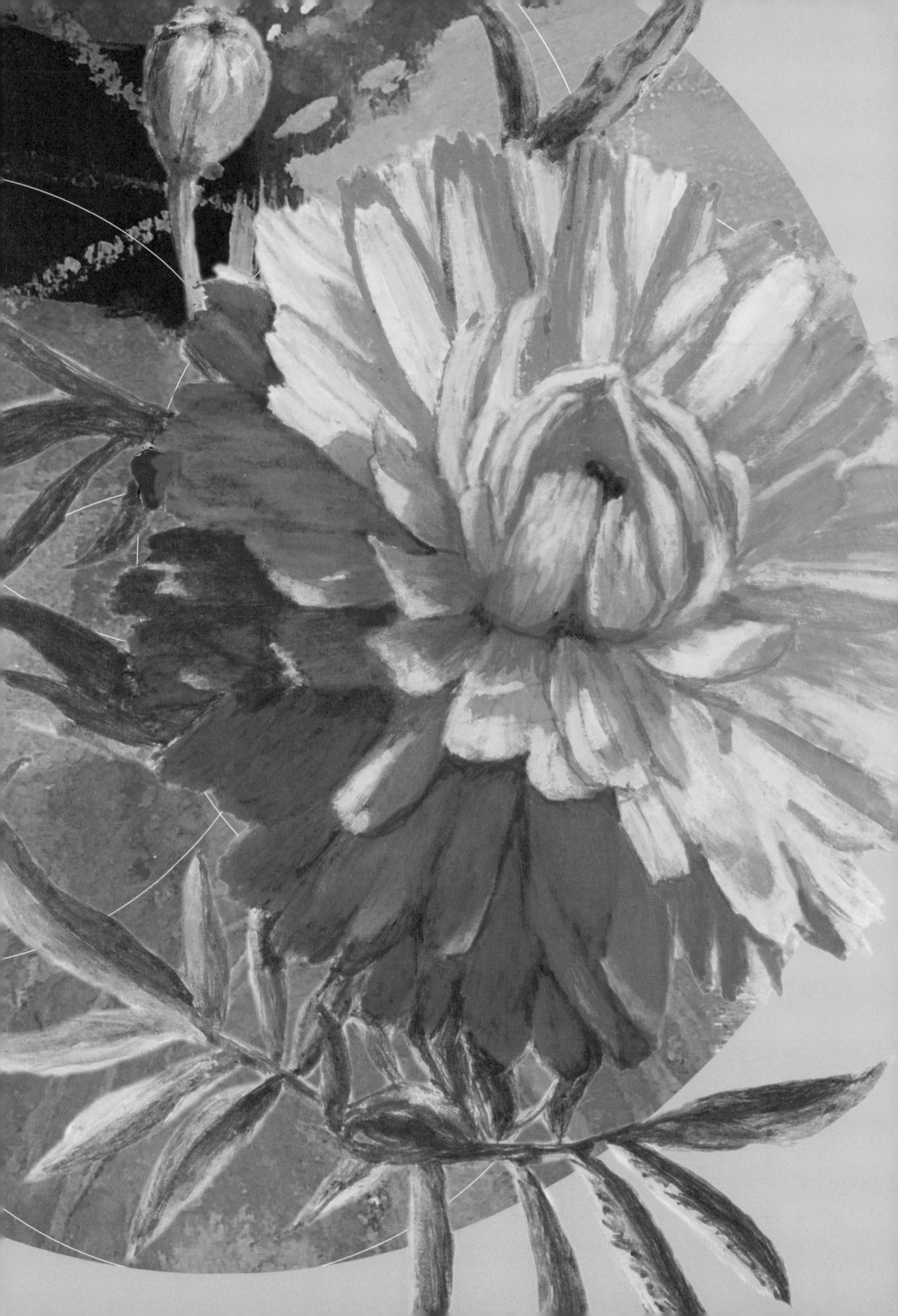

9 Flower Essences for Frustration

"

If you so choose, every mistake can lead to greater understanding and effectiveness. If you so choose, every frustration can help you to be more patient and more persistent.

— Ralph Marston

Frustration can arise easily when your needs are not being met—whether you, others, or even societal structures are to blame. When you feel frustrated, it is easy to grow more reactive in your emotions and be drawn out of center. You may have heard that anger can be a cover-up for sadness or grief. Indeed, if we allow anger or frustration to pass within us without clinging to it, we may notice that there is a grief or somberness behind it. It is important to feel and recognize the subtler layers in our emotional body so that we can integrate them from a place of witnessing. Often emotional reactions come from early childhood experiences not yet fully integrated and realized. Through a variety of practices, you can allow for your full range of emotions and embody more peace. Frustration serves a purpose; it can be a sign that you should make a change, for example. Once you are in a calmer or more centered state, you can take action to meet the needs that were not being met before. So in the end, your frustration can be a gift for transformation.

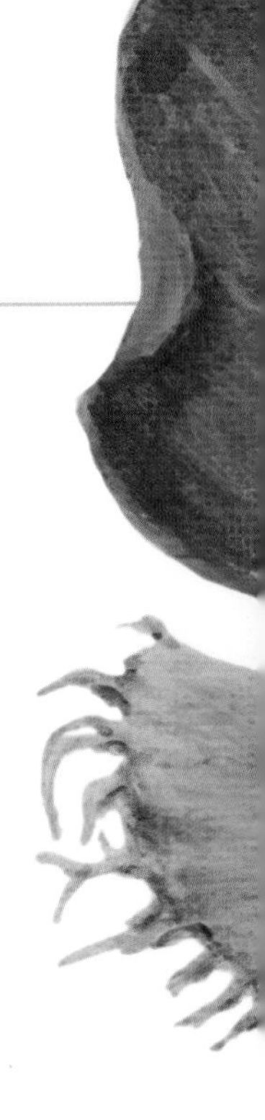

Beech

BEECH FLOWER ESSENCE WILL ASSIST YOU WITH:

- Easing judgment of others
- Alleviating frustration
- Becoming more open-minded

Invocation

Take Beech flower essence with you the next time you go out in public. Sit at a café or some other place where you can people-watch. Notice if any judgments toward others arise. Now take the essence and see if that criticism subsides.

Native to temperate parts of Asia, Europe, and North America, Beech is a deciduous tree that is monoecious, meaning it has both male and female flowers on the same plant. The flower essence is an important healer for those who are often in a fixed mental state and critical or intolerant of others. Beech can assist in alleviating dissatisfaction and irritability within, especially when looking at people outside oneself. Someone who would benefit from taking this essence may often need strict order and could be overly disciplined. Beech brings about a more flexible and fluid state in which one can accept others—and oneself—with more love and understanding. A more balanced and positive outlook toward life is also a gift of this essence. If you often find yourself criticizing others in your mind, allow Beech to transform you from a rigid state into openness and acceptance.

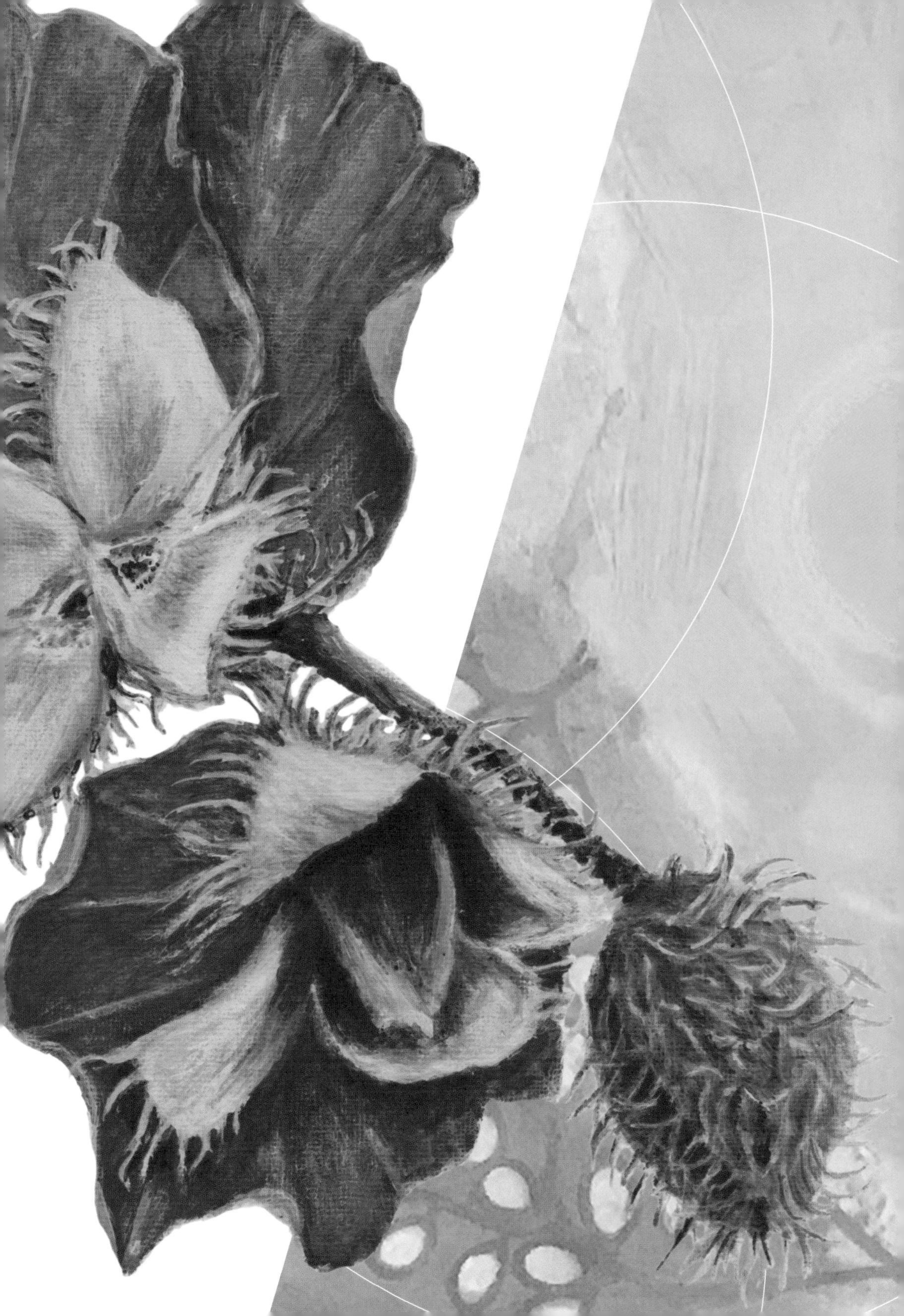

Calendula

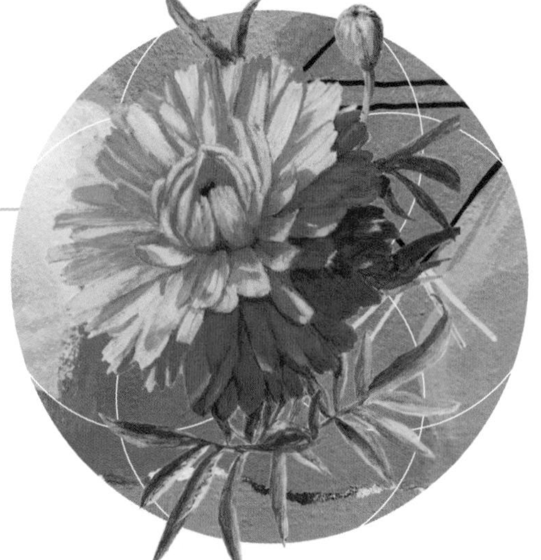

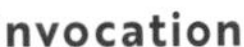

CALENDULA FLOWER ESSENCE WILL ASSIST YOU WITH:

- Releasing angry verbal reactions
- Inspiring more warmth and receptivity
- Cultivating empathy and radiance

Invocation

Grab a blanket, go outdoors, and lie in the sunshine. Take Calendula flower essence and feel the warmth of the light permeate your body, particularly your throat and solar plexus chakras. The healing power of this essence can transform patterns of verbal abuse or anger into more empathy and receptivity to others.

Belonging to the daisy family, this herbaceous plant is native to the Mediterranean, Macaronesia, and Asia. Often known as marigold, it is used for its medicinal properties. Calendula flower essence is an energetic healer for those who tend to be argumentative and express frustration or anger verbally. The soothing and bright qualities of this essence bring about lightness and radiance within, opening up channels of receptivity and warmth. Calendula transforms pent-up feelings of frustration into understanding and empathy for both the self and others. Communication becomes more authentic and heartfelt. Because it is also a healer of the solar plexus chakra, feelings of self-acceptance and self-worth may also increase. Overall, Calendula is a magick maker when you desire more light-filled experiences inside yourself and in relation to others.

Fuchsia

FUCHSIA FLOWER ESSENCE WILL ASSIST YOU WITH:

- Balancing out intense emotional states
- Embracing suppressed anger and grief
- Expressing feelings authentically

Invocation

Take this flower essence and turn on some music (perhaps a sentimental, cathartic dance track), loudly if you wish. Shake, shake, shake, and dance out pent-up feelings! Cry, scream, laugh, and roll around on the floor—do whatever you need to do to release suppressed emotions. Notice how Fuchsia supports you in this surrender.

Native to parts of South and Central America, this plant is part of a genus that consists of highly decorative flowering shrubs and small trees. Fuchsia flower essence is an apropos healer for those who have an intensely suppressed range of emotions, including trauma. Sometimes life can be so challenging that when painful occurrences take place, it can be too much to process fully and a soul, out of its own protection, represses them. The problem is that those repressed feelings and memories then affect our subconscious, and soon our habitual ways of reacting to life may not best serve as well as they could. This flower essence helps free up those emotions, thus making space in the core being and allowing access to the repressed parts. If you often find yourself covering up your real feelings while being deeply affected by them when alone, Fuchsia is a perfect medicine for you. This essence allows for authenticity and a healthy life full of feeling—one that is liberated, courageous, and in tune with the subtle layers of the emotional body.

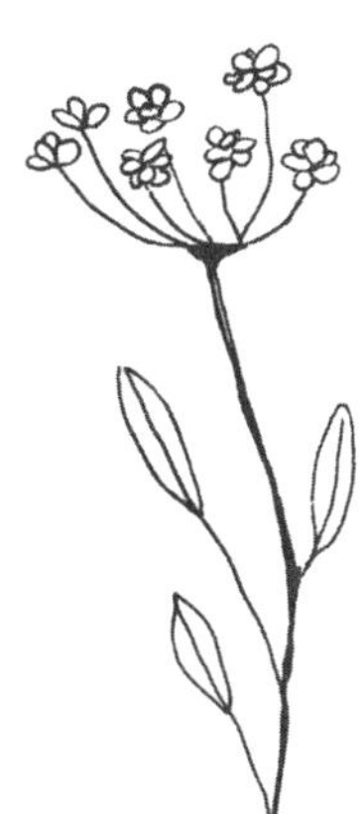

Hawthorn

HAWTHORN FLOWER ESSENCE WILL ASSIST YOU WITH:

- Freeing up agitation and stress
- Balancing out a forceful will
- Inspiring heartfelt courage

Invocation

Find a quiet place to sit and meditate and take this flower essence. Take this time to be with your heart. Place both hands over your heart and allow all your attention and focus, including your breath, to travel to it. Attention is love; it cools and eases feelings of stress. Breathe into your heart. Allow your breath to nourish and let Hawthorn flower essence work its magick.

Belonging to the family Rosaceae, this genus contains several hundred species of shrubs and small trees. The berry is often used as an herbal medicine for heart, digestive, or circulatory issues. Hawthorn flower essence, however, can help when someone's personality turns to a habitual state of hostility or aggression. When this happens, the vitality of the heart's love forces has been depleted, and the person may find him- or herself with an overworked strong will or forceful disposition. Hawthorn flower essence can alleviate such symptoms and help bring more balance into these energy centers (specifically the solar plexus and heart chakra). After taking this essence, a forceful will transforms into courageous action that is led from the heart. A more positive outlook can be instilled. The physical body is inspired to do good, from a place of power that is led more by love and less by the need for control. Take Hawthorn if you wish to have your place of will integrated with the place of love within you.

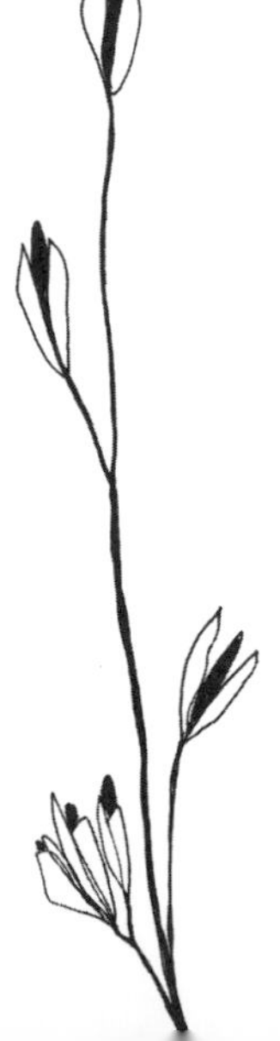

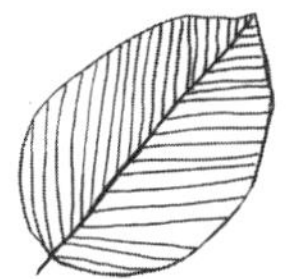

Holly

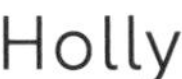

HOLLY FLOWER ESSENCE WILL ASSIST YOU WITH:

- Absolving jealousy and anger
- Opening up the heart
- Dropping into compassion and universal love

Invocation

Take Holly flower essence and sit outside to people-watch. Breathe into your heart and imagine it opening up to the universal law and flow of love that runs though you and all things. Notice your heart opening and feeling more empathy for the world. Today is a new day to love more fully.

An evergreen tree or shrub that's native to Europe as well as parts of Africa and Asia, Holly has long been celebrated during the Christmas season, when it features prominently in holiday decorations from wreaths to garlands. Holly flower essence allows us to feel love in a bigger way than before, tapping into the flow of love through the universe and in all sentient beings. It also assists in alleviating envy, jealousy, and even anger. If you find yourself easily becoming suspicious of others and thus frustrated, Holly is a pertinent healer for you. It restores in the soul a sense of connection and unity, to oneself and to others. From there compassion can grow, and one can return to a feeling of being held in universal love and benevolence. This flower essence is a true tonic for the heart chakra; it expands it to feel saturated with divinity and goodwill. Holly takes us from frustration to wholeness, a true blessing indeed.

Impatiens

IMPATIENS FLOWER ESSENCE WILL ASSIST YOU WITH:

- Clearing impatience and intolerance
- Bestowing acceptance
- Inspiring patience and depth to the soul

Invocation

Take this flower essence with you for a walk into nature. After imbibing it, slow down to stroll and notice how nature flows and dances with life. Allow this energy to inspire you and help release pent-up feelings of anger. Allow your mind and heart to open up. Breathe in patience and acceptance. Embodying these two virtues will truly transform your life.

Native to the Himalayan region, this annual plant can grow up to 6 feet (1.8 m) high with hat-shaped flowers. Impatiens flower essence is beneficial to individuals who are intolerant and easily frustrated in life. This could be because the awareness and gift of the present moment are often ignored, as these souls feel a need to rush through life in a frantic and anxious state. When doing so, the preciousness and soft quality of the moment are overlooked. Impatiens assists in allowing patience to be restored. It provides a sense of peace and acceptance for what is taking place now. Irritation shifts to calm; impatience and tension transform into receptivity and awareness. The breath deepens, slows down, and appreciates the passage of time and the splendor of life in all its beauty.

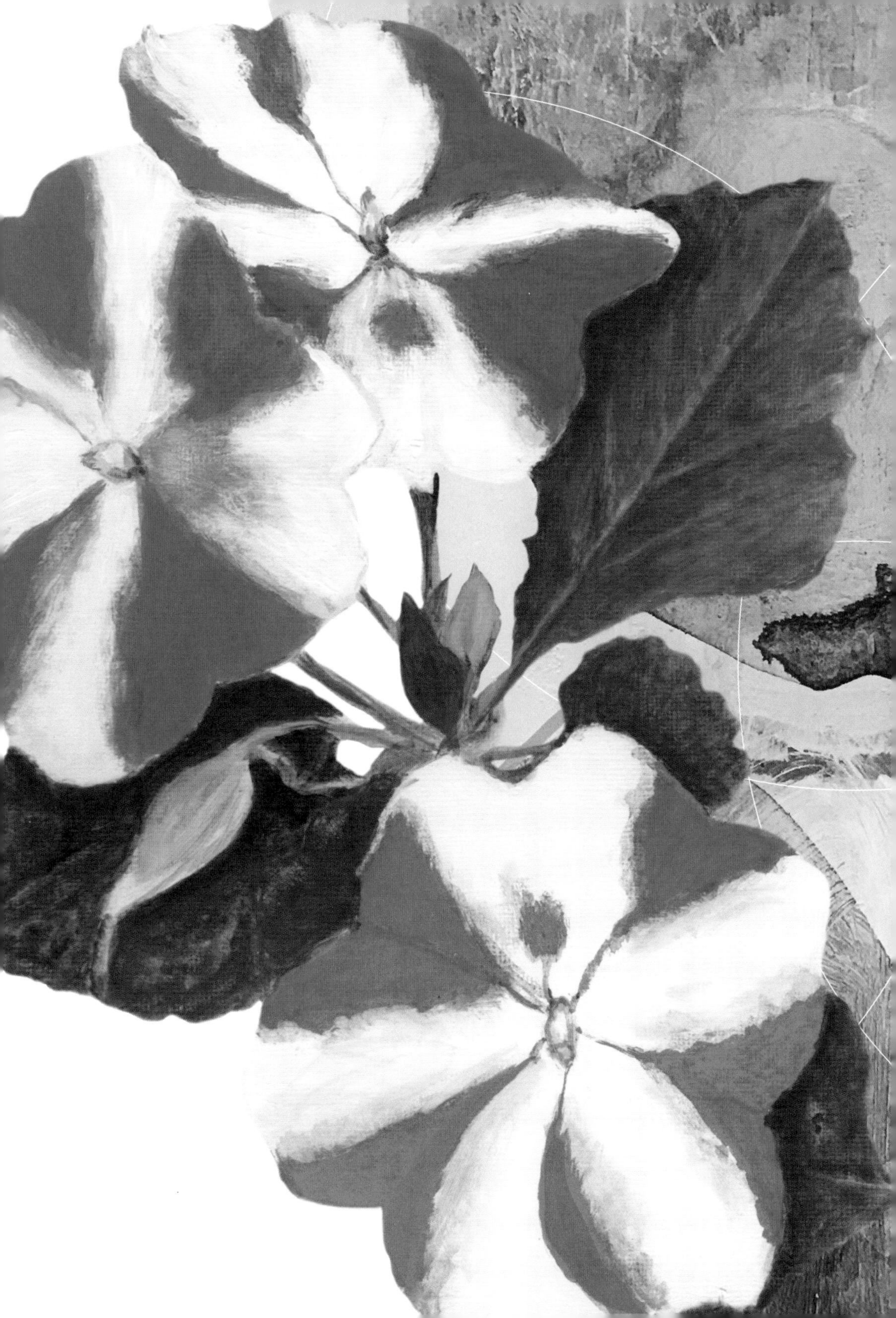

Ocotillo

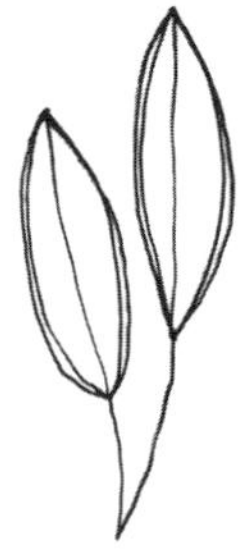

OCOTILLO FLOWER ESSENCE WILL ASSIST YOU WITH:

- Discharging anger and volatility
- Clearing up projections
- Integrating fiery tendencies into heart-based energy

Invocation

Take this flower essence before you shower, bathe, or go out for a swim. As you enter the water, envision how the energetic properties of Ocotillo also cool your internal flames. The gift of this essence is that deep anger is mutated into feelings of love and acceptance. Let it provide these much-needed states within you.

Also known as Candlewood or Desert Coral, this plant blooms with crimson flowers after a good rainfall and is native to the southwestern United States. Ocotillo is a valuable flower essence for those who feel highly imbalanced and have feelings of anger and reactivity to others. A soul who often projects suppressed emotions, and thus reacts in frustrated and intolerant ways, would benefit from taking this flower essence. Ocotillo drops the energy down into one's center and heart, thus transforming into a core feeling of radiance. This flower essence helps soothe such fires within, inviting a response of clarity to situations rather than overreaction. It inspires a sense of security and love for yourself, which makes interacting with others much smoother. This flower essence also brings about a feeling of protection and well-being, and thus defensive walls are dismantled. Invite Ocotillo into your life if you are going through a period of anger and even emotional volatility, and see how much relief it provides.

Tiger Lily

TIGER LILY FLOWER ESSENCE WILL ASSIST YOU WITH:

- Dissolving frustration and hostility
- Transforming aggression into receptivity
- Inspiring inner peace and harmony with others

Invocation

Take this flower essence with you to a natural body of water, such as a river, pond, lake, or creek. Take the essence while noticing the flowing, receptive state of the water. See how it flows with life, not against it. Tiger Lily can shift your frustration into calm, just like the effortless nature of the water.

Native to the southwestern part of the United States and Baja, Mexico, this orange-spotted lily gloriously flowers in the month of June. Tiger Lily flower essence is an essential healer for those who tend to have excessive masculine or yang forces, which can range from overcompetitiveness to hostility and aggression. The energetic medicine of this essence grants a feeling of service and cooperation with others. Tiger Lily inspires more feminine, or yin, qualities, such as heightened sensitivity and understanding when relating. This essence also provides a desire to work with others in acts of service for the greater good. A balance of both yin and yang energies takes place, providing for more integrated relationships with all. Take Tiger Lily if you feel frustrated within and competitive with fellow humans; see how a sense of harmony and cooperation is bestowed instead.

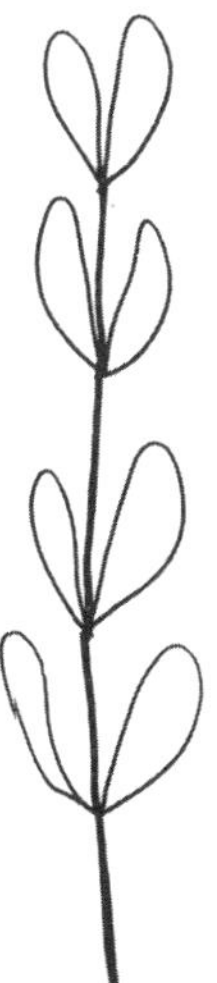

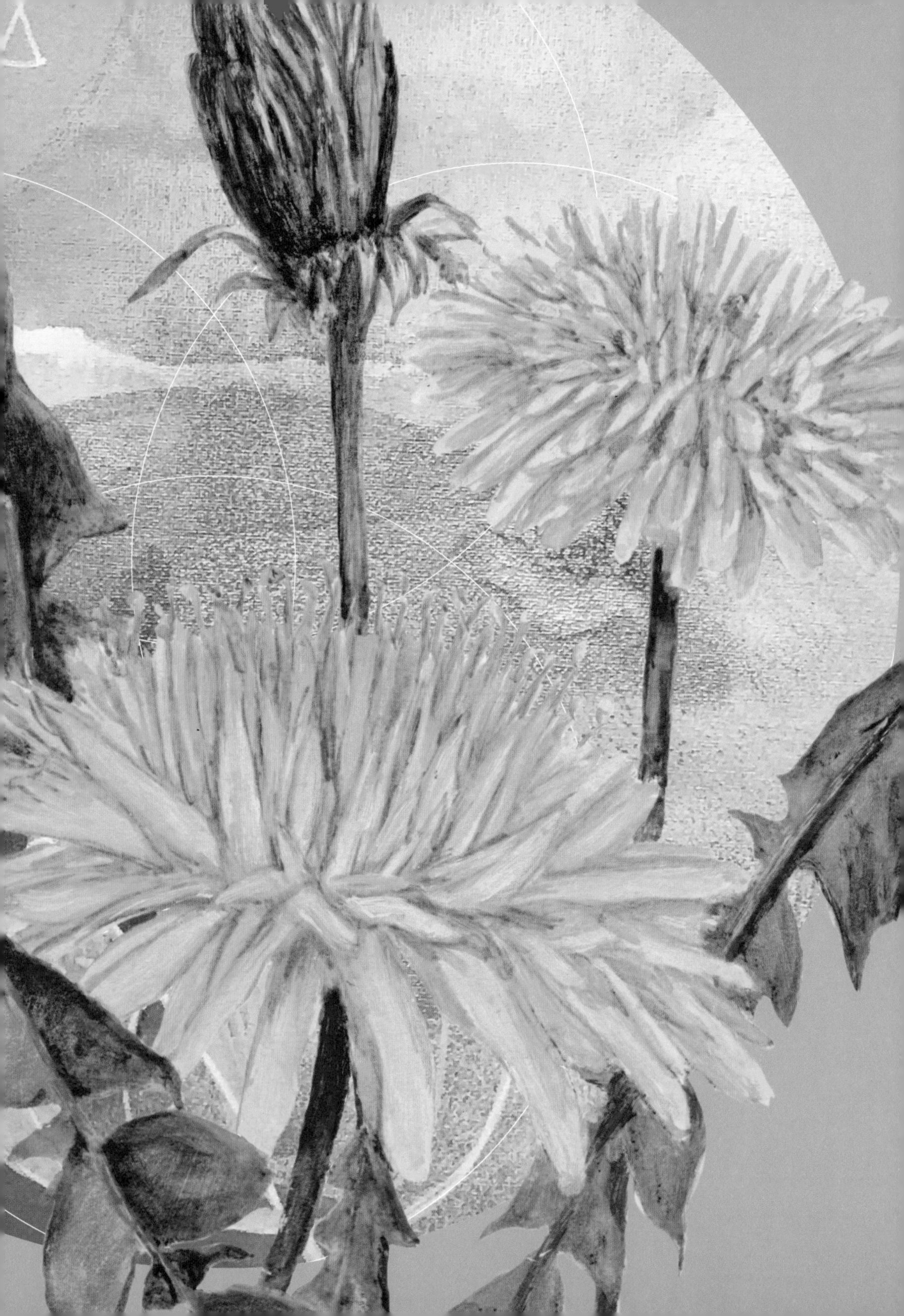

10 Flower Essences for Grounding

"

The highest levels of performance come to people who are centered, intuitive, creative, and reflective—people who know to see a problem as an opportunity.

—Deepak Chopra

In a world that is always "on," it's imperative to stay grounded and centered inside the core of yourself. If we have daily practices to ground our energies within as well as get in touch with nature, life flows more gracefully. Those practices can be meditation, *pranayama* or breath work, martial arts (especially ones that connect breath to movement), long walks, artistic endeavors, yoga, journaling, or the like. The art of ritual also helps us ground ourselves. It's become apparent that the Western world has forgotten the practice of ceremony, even though coming together as a community in the spirit of ritual helps ground the collective. Fortunately, we have the flower essences in this chapter to help us stay grounded. As above, so below . . . may you walk gently upon the path and feel the connectedness of all things. May you know how the earth and flowers are here to support and inspire you.

Almond

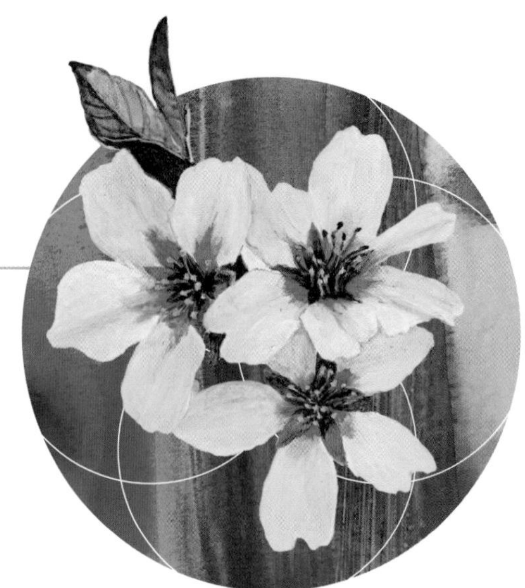

ALMOND FLOWER ESSENCE WILL ASSIST YOU WITH:

- Finding balance over excess
- Releasing negative habits
- Residing in a place of calm

Invocation

Take Almond flower essence and spend the day slowing down and noticing details. Every hour, stop and breathe deeply with your eyes closed for a few minutes. Notice how this essence allows you to unfold each day in a natural rhythm, trusting that all will get done more easily from a place of centeredness.

The Almond tree, cultivated in many places around the world, yet native to Iran and central Asia, grows up to 33 feet (10 m) in height. Its flowers are pink and white, bloom in spring, and do best in temperate climates. This flower essence assists us in grounding nervous energy or overindulgent activities so that we feel balanced. If you find yourself overworking, staying busy to stay busy, partaking in addictive patterns of excess, and becoming easily frustrated, then Almond could be your ally. Almond helps relax the body and quiet the mind, so that life flows rather than feeling forced. Excessive heat may cool in the body, and moderation becomes a value for the soul who takes this ancient essence. Receive the gift of the Almond flower essence to restore healthy practices and balance in the energetic bodies.

Blackberry

BLACKBERRY FLOWER ESSENCE WILL ASSIST YOU WITH:

- Staying on task with goals
- Embodying decisiveness
- Manifesting with ease

Invocation

Go outside with this flower essence and walk barefoot on the earth. Say the following affirmation to yourself as you take Blackberry: "I stay focused on my path and manifest ideas with ease and flow." A new way of actualizing your dreams is now afoot!

Native to the western part of North America, this wild berry feeds many animals and is an essential pollinator for bees. Native Americans have used it as a medicinal plant, and it is used widely as an edible fruit. The pink and white flowers of this essence are incredibly helpful to those who struggle to stay on track with realizing goals. If you find yourself easily distracted with too many ideas and not enough willpower to make your dreams happen, then Blackberry is for you. This powerful little essence helps you stay grounded while taking viable action to reach your goals every day. It assists in the manifestation process of actualizing dreams by filling you with enthusiasm and clarity. Awaken to the power you hold within and allow Blackberry to be your ally along the way.

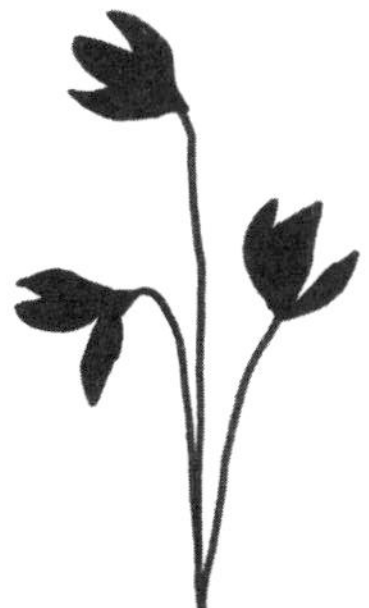

Clematis

CLEMATIS FLOWER ESSENCE WILL ASSIST YOU WITH:

- Balancing daydreaming
- Embodying presence in the now
- Attaining goals every day

Invocation

Go outside and take off your shoes. Walk barefoot on the earth and feel how Gaia supports you. Take this flower essence and sit down in a comfortable place. Notice how your energy begins to ground. Breathe into the here and now and feel your awareness growing inside the present moment. This is the gift of Clematis.

Native to England and Asia, this beautiful flower comes in a variety of colors and is a deciduous, fast-climbing shrub that blooms in the summer. Its seeds have long, feathered tails. The flower essence of Clematis is perfect for creative dreamers filled with many longings and aspirations, especially if they often get lost thinking about the future instead of being in the present moment. These individuals struggle when dealing with reality as it is now. It is also helpful for those who are often caught daydreaming yet struggle to actualize their dreams in real life. Clematis helps heal those who feel ungrounded, with their head in the clouds. It centers them so they fully become aware of the gifts alive in front of them, and it helps manifest their dreams by focusing on the tangible actions that are steps toward them. Take this flower essence if you often project yourself into the future and wish to regain your center to begin making your aspirations a reality.

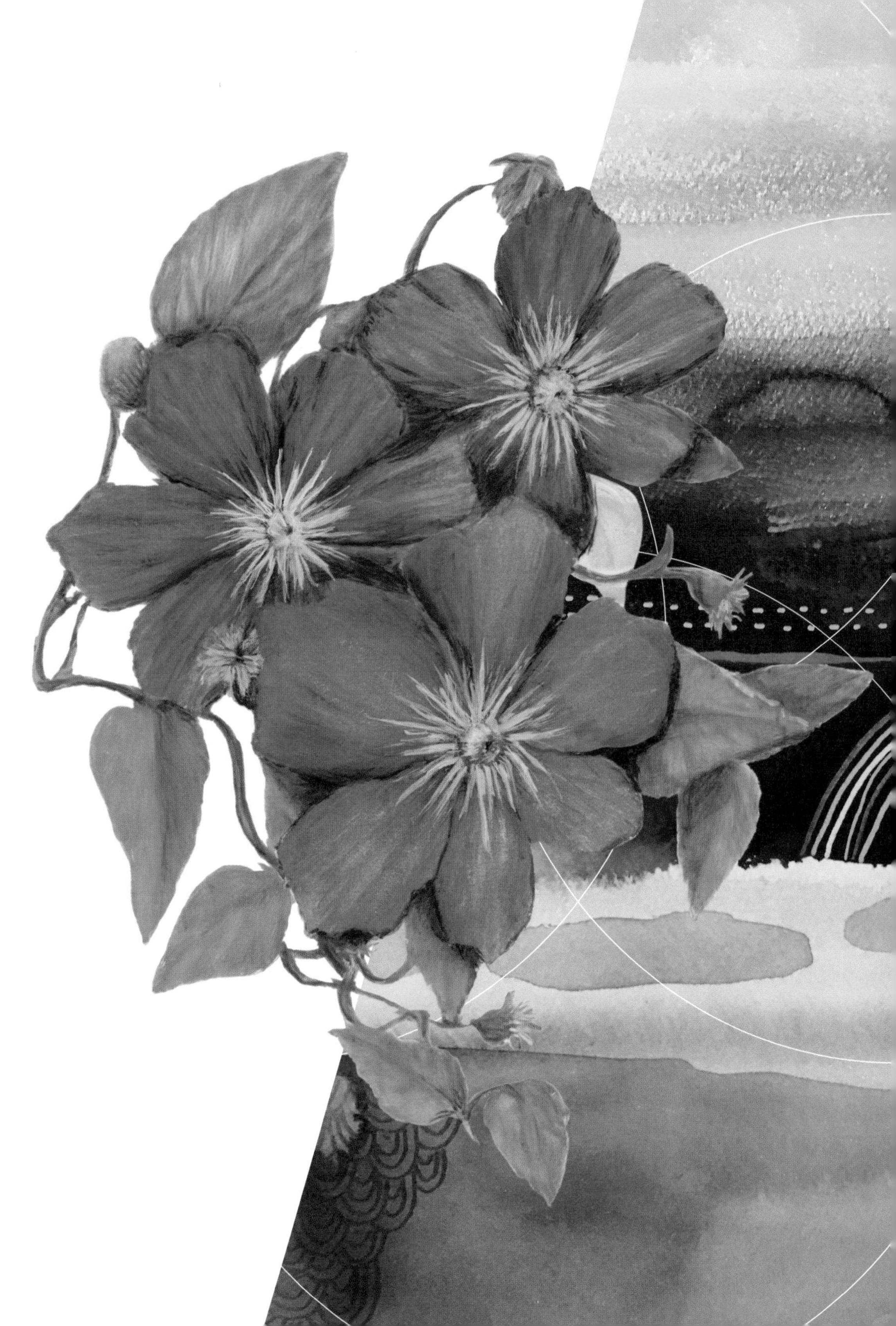

Dandelion

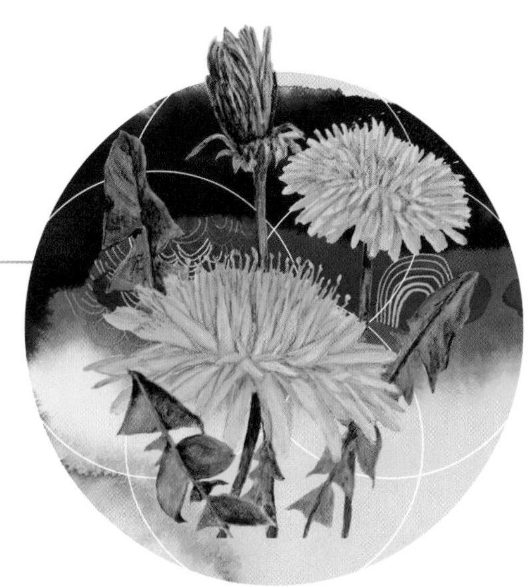

DANDELION FLOWER ESSENCE WILL ASSIST YOU WITH:

- Alleviating tense ambition
- Relaxing the muscular structure
- Revitalizing the dynamic and universal life force

Invocation

Take this flower essence and then allow some quiet moments to stretch out your whole body. Consider attending a restorative yoga class afterward. Notice how you feel awake, revitalized, and full of energy the next morning. This is how Dandelion works its magick.

This powerful flower, more commonly known for its herbal medicinal qualities, can be found all over the world in temperate climates. It grows along highways, in lawns, at shores of water, and elsewhere. Dandelion flower essence assists in healing a tense muscular-skeletal system, one that has been working too hard and been tense for too long. This alleviating yet rejuvenating essence helps relax that tension and brings the energy and focus back in the universal life force that runs through us all. Physical vitality is restored again and feels more effortless. If you have been burning the candle at both ends and driving yourself to exhaustion, Dandelion will help bring you back into your center of balance. Feelings of resentment toward family and other people are also alleviated. Tasks begin to complete themselves with ease instead of strife. The many gifts of Dandelion help heal an overworked and tense human family, which is perhaps why this mighty plant is found so plentifully all over the world.

Lady's Slipper

LADY'S SLIPPER FLOWER ESSENCE WILL ASSIST YOU WITH:

- Alleviating anxious energy
- Becoming more grounded with your spiritual self
- Finding true purpose with work

Invocation

Find a quiet place to sit, reflect, and meditate and take this flower essence. Feel how your lower energy centers or chakras vibrate all the way up to the crown chakra or top of your head. Breathe in and feel the integration of all your energy as one. Lady's Slipper helps us balance and find our way with purpose.

Native to North America, this orchid flower is widespread throughout the United States and grows in a variety of habitats, from damp and coniferous forests to open meadows and streams. The flower essence of Lady's Slipper is unique in its purpose of healing. It assists the soul in becoming more unified in all its energy centers, from the base or root chakra to the crown chakra. People who would benefit from taking this essence often do not realize their true gifts in life and therefore their vocation does not reflect their soul purpose and authentic desires. Lady's Slipper helps center your energy so that you can realize your unique power and capabilities and just how to walk your path in this world. This flower essence eases nervous tension and revitalizes sensual or sexual vitality. It may ignite the intuition and guidance from feeling more integrated and connected to the earth and to all parts of being. Lady's Slipper bestows a sense of calm, unity, and security and thus can inspire you to feel creative and put you back on your path of purpose in this life.

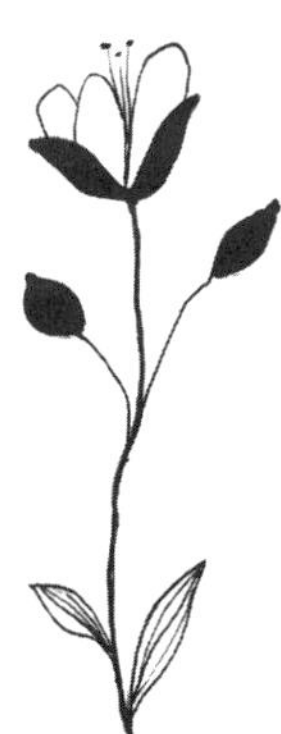

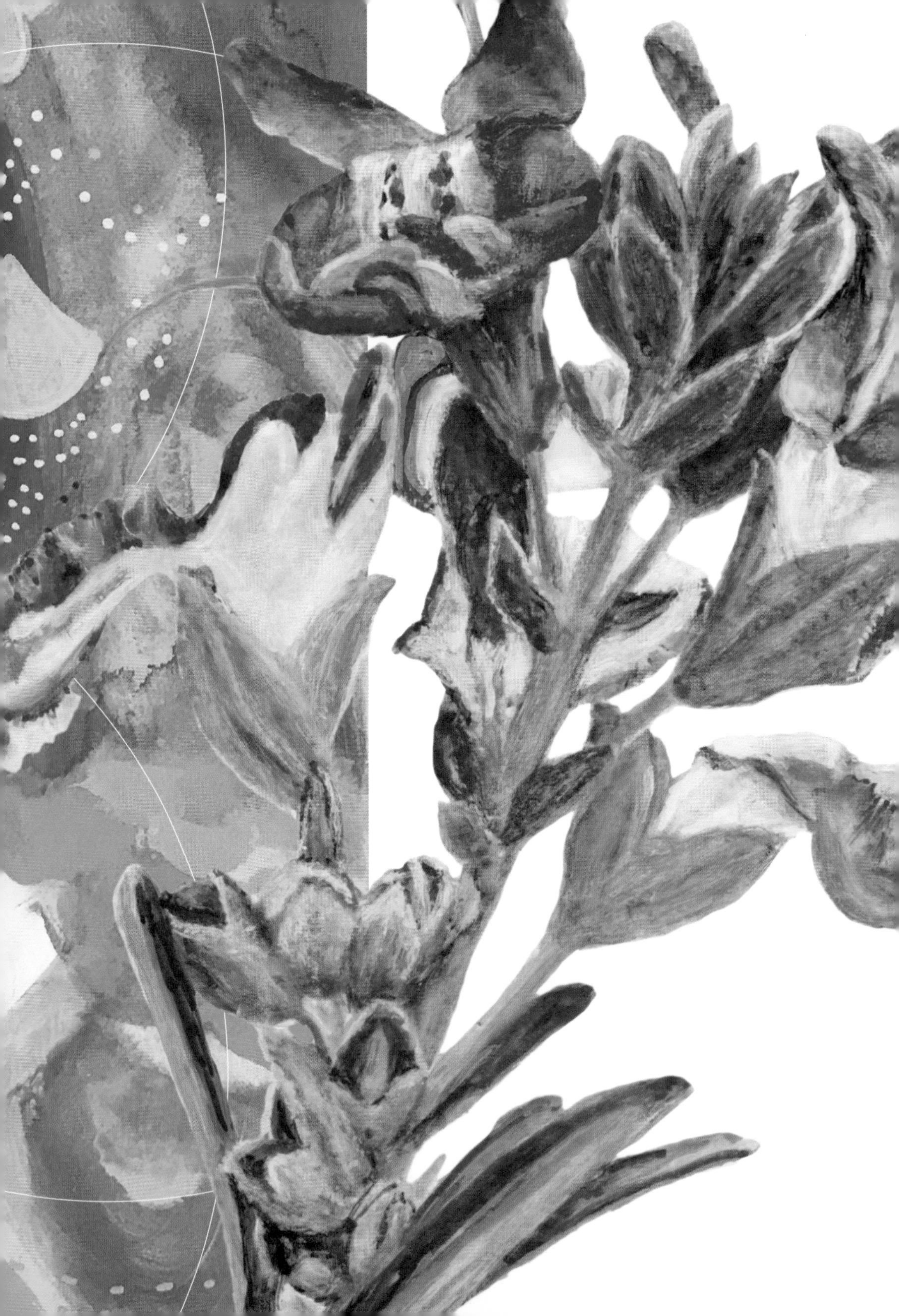

Rosemary

ROSEMARY FLOWER ESSENCE WILL ASSIST YOU WITH:

- Easing melancholy and depression
- Feeling motivated and inspired
- Grounding you with resilience and calm

Invocation

Put on an outfit that makes you feel beautiful. Take Rosemary flower essence and allow your soul to dance. Feelings of rejuvenation, joy, and a zest for living may return. You have been forewarned!

An evergreen native to the Mediterranean and a member of the mint family Lamiaceae, this herbaceous plant is known best for its aromatic and flavorful qualities when used in cooking. The petal blooms are white, pink, or bluish purple. As a flower essence, it is restorative—joyful yet grounding. Rosemary reminds you to feel enthusiasm for living life here and now on earth. It awakens emotional balance and a calm feeling in the energy systems of the body. And it gives you a vital and whole feeling of the physical body. Poor memory and lack of focus are assuaged. This powerful essence can help integrate your physical and emotional states in numerous ways, if you allow her. Give yourself the gift of Rosemary when a zest for living from a grounded place is calling you.

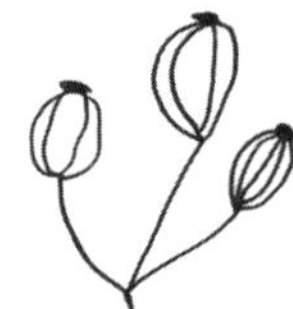

Sweet Pea

SWEET PEA FLOWER ESSENCE WILL ASSIST YOU WITH:

- Healing feelings of uprootedness or an inability to find home
- Connecting more deeply to community
- Feeling a place of grounded belonging on earth

Invocation

Sit under a tree and breathe deeply into your base or root chakra (near the perineum or just below the spine). Take Sweet Pea flower essence and feel your energy grounding into Mother Earth. Feel yourself being held gently. If you are feeling lost without a place to call home, envision where you desire your true home to be. Allow the energy of this essence to carry you there.

A climbing plant with darling flowers that come in a variety of pastel shades, Sweet Pea is native to Sicily, southern Italy, and the Aegean Islands. Sweet Pea flower essence is extremely helpful for those who are feeling lost with no place to call home. It can also provide energetic assistance if you have made a commitment to a place but can't connect to others in the area or cultivate community or friendships. Sweet Pea flower essence eases feelings of disconnection and isolation, and it inspires bonds with others while you form a stronger foundation within yourself. Deeper and more authentic connections are formed with others, within yourself, and with the feeling of home here on Earth. Sweet pea helps balance the root chakra and provides vitality and sweetness in trusting being alive here and now.

Vervain

VERVAIN FLOWER ESSENCE WILL ASSIST YOU WITH:

- Assuaging perfectionism
- Easing the need to constantly be persuasive
- Enjoying life in the moment

Invocation

Look in the mirror right when you wake up and notice all the details of your face and body. Notice if any critical feelings or mental chatter come up. Take this flower essence and relax into the energies of acceptance and allowance, along with your desire to persuade others into your way of thinking. You are perfect just as you are.

Native to parts of Europe, this perennial herb with purplish-blue flowers has a rich folkloric history for its healing and herbal medicine properties. Vervain flower essence assists in alleviating a need to heavily convert others to your way of thinking, no matter what the cause or desire is. This can come from a need for perfection or from constant mental chatter about how things ought to be. Fixed personalities who often feel they are right can benefit from taking Vervain. If you notice any of these qualities in yourself, this essence may be (ironically) the perfect healer for you. Allow yourself to ground into the beauty of the moment as it is right now, without the need to persuade or do anything, but simply to enjoy reality as it is.

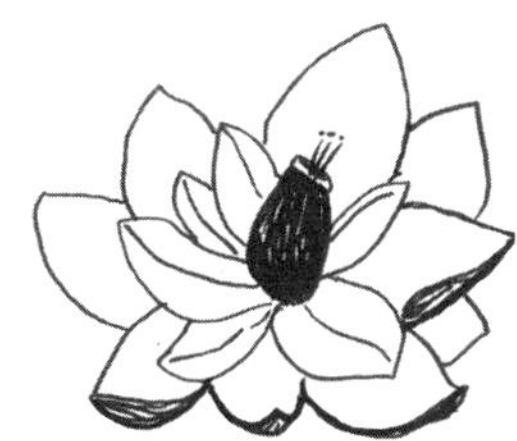

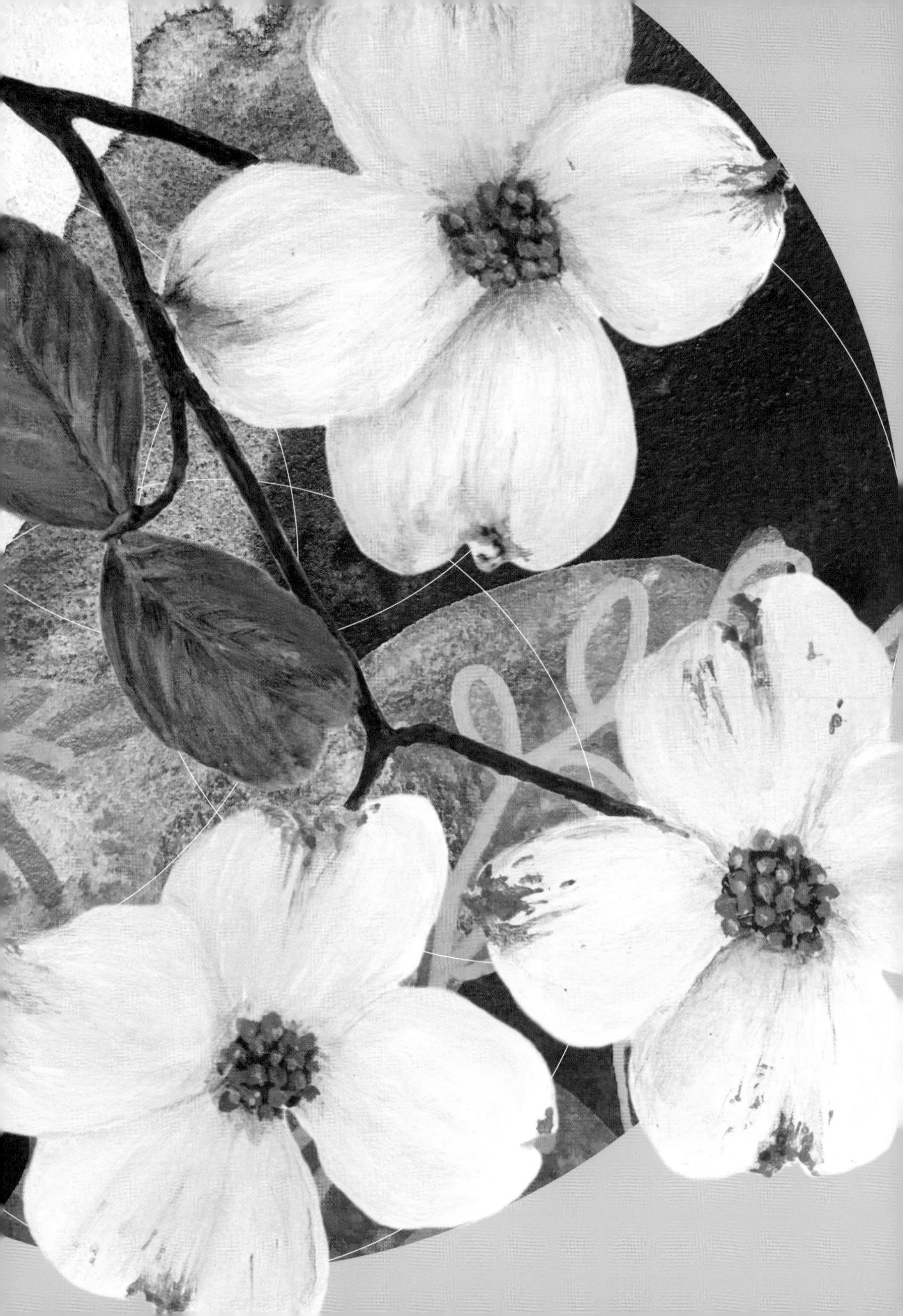

11 Flower Essences for Healing

"

Confront the dark parts of yourself, and work to banish them with illumination and forgiveness. Your willingness to wrestle with your demons will cause your angels to sing.

— *August Wilson*

When our soul decides to enter a body, it's as if we are entering a contract for our own accelerated healing and integration of all parts of our being. And being in "Earth school" is no laughing matter: Much healing is needed on the planet right now, and much of it starts with the consciousness of human beings. We have immense capabilities of transformation through our own practices, so how can we become more aware and whole so that we live a life of harmony with each other, the earth, and ourselves? What essential tools do we need to allow this healing to take place? How can we arrive fully in our bodies with a clear mind and live through and from the heart? We are exploring many of these questions right now. Let the flower essences listed below also be an integral part of your journey.

Arnica

ARNICA FLOWER ESSENCE WILL ASSIST YOU WITH:

- Healing from shock or disassociated states
- Sparking recovery from trauma
- Instilling a centered connection or embodiment

Invocation

Take your Arnica flower essence and put on your favorite music, preferably something that is calming and healing in nature. Wrap yourself in a warm blanket if you wish. Lie down in a comfortable place and feel this essence moving through all your energy. Allow this unwinding to take place.

A part of the sunflower family, this perennial herb, which has yellow flowers, is native to Canada and parts of the United States. Arnica flower essence is best used when traumatic events have caused intense shock. When such events occur, pain can get stuck in the body and the subconscious, so it's important to allow this healing and release to take place consciously and with a lot of care. This potent essence is all about experiencing a substantial recovery. When you take Arnica, the consciousness comes back into union with the whole self, so that the protected parts of the self that have shut down can be activated again. Sometimes this process can be quite intense, so be sure to reach out to groups or a professional (such as a somatic therapist) who can help that alignment happen with more ease and grace.

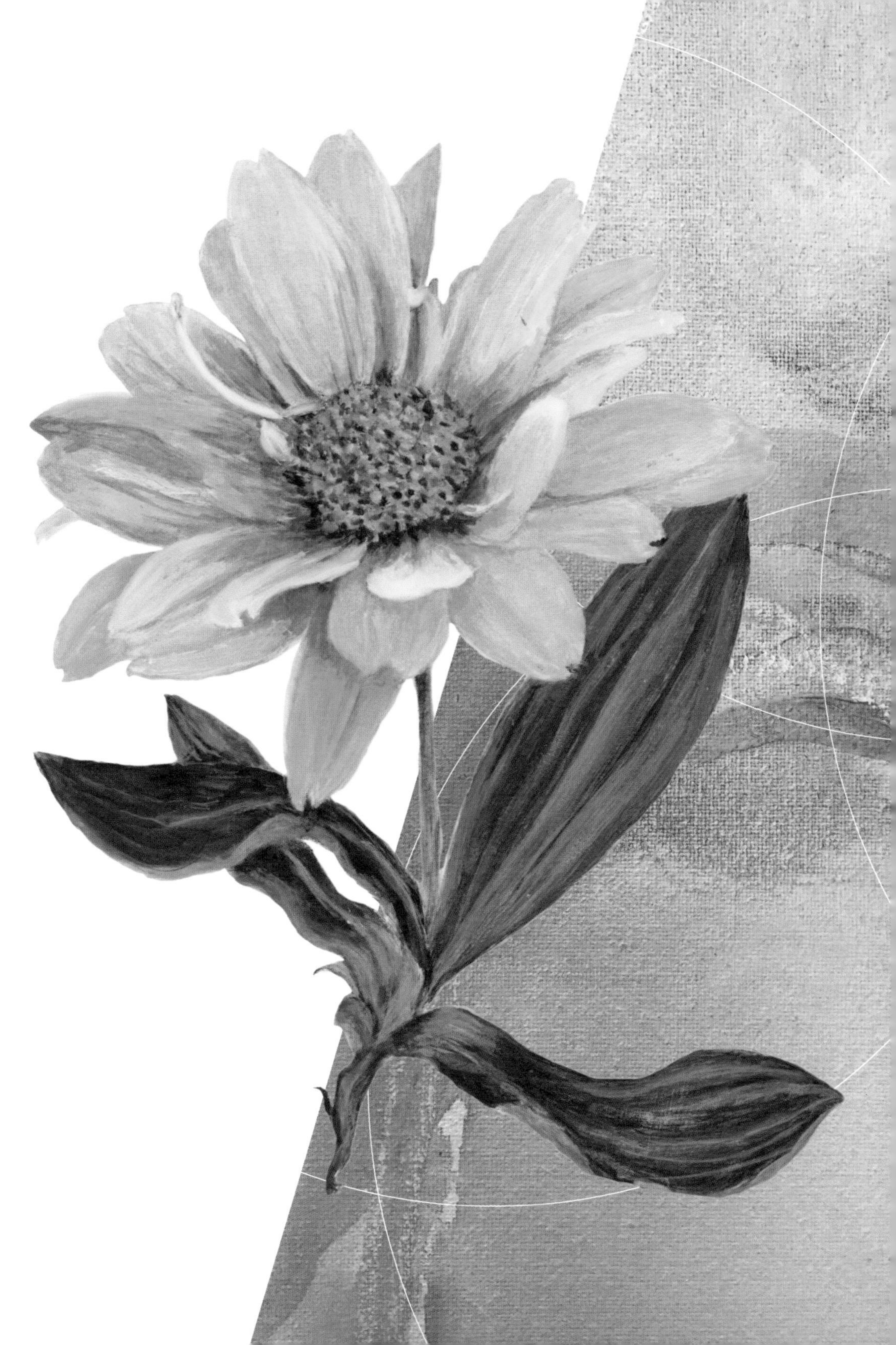

Crab Apple

CRAB APPLE FLOWER ESSENCE WILL ASSIST YOU WITH:

- Alleviating obsessive tendencies
- Releasing the need for perfection
- Inspiring a sense of purity

Invocation

Grab a journal and make a list of all the negative things about yourself that you tend to obsess about. You can also add things about your life or the world in general—include anything about which you can feel your perfectionism or need for control becoming activated. Take Crab Apple flower essence. After the list is complete, burn it or dissolve it in water and bury it. Say aloud, "Today I let go of my inner critic and need for perfection."

Native to Europe, this bush-like tree can live for up to one hundred years. Its name means "forest apple." The flower essence of the Crab Apple, with its white flowers touched with a bit of pink, is for those who often feel unclean. If you tend to be obsessive about achieving perfection, which can often be the result of layers of shame underneath, this could be a very helpful flower essence. Viewing oneself critically can often start with the physical body, then encompass how one keeps house and so forth. A need for cleanliness and order becomes paramount, to the point of taking away fulfillment from daily life. Crab Apple inspires balance within and helps lessen a compulsive need to feel clean. After taking this essence, remember that imperfection is a necessary part of the journey, and one's true purity comes from within, in relationship to oneself.

Dogwood

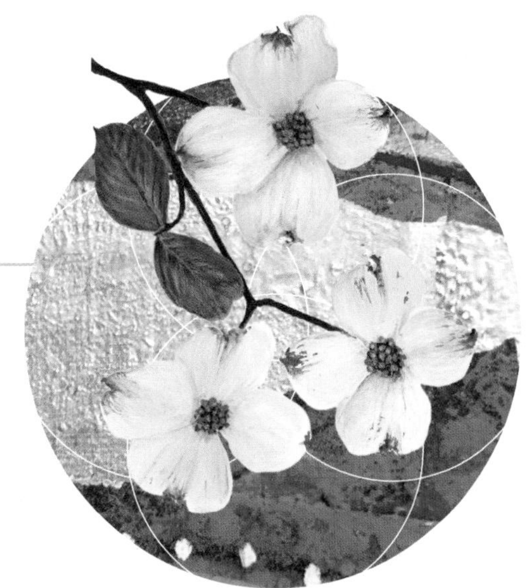

DOGWOOD FLOWER ESSENCE WILL ASSIST YOU WITH:

- Easing stiffness in the body
- Clearing emotional trauma
- Encouraging graceful movement and harmony

Invocation

Take Dogwood flower essence and then attend a restorative yoga class or gently stretch for some time at home. Breathe deeply into the tense parts of your body. Afterward, soak in a hot bath with Epsom salts. Envision your body unwinding deeply. Do this routine daily (plus whatever else to support your healing) until you begin to feel peace in your physical form.

A medium-size deciduous tree with small white flowers that can grow up to 80 feet (24.4 m) tall, the Dogwood is native to British Columbia and western parts of the United States. Dogwood flower essence can help when repeated trauma or emotional hardship has been suppressed in the physical form. This happens when protected layers form within the body and it becomes stiff, tense, and inflexible. This can result in pain and loss of grace in movement. This flower essence is appropriate if you are feeling a lack of harmony in your body and longing for union and softness within. Take the essence regularly and supplement it with other methods of support to heal yourself and alleviate the pain. Massage therapy, yoga, hot baths with salt, and physical therapy are just some of the modalities you can try. You may also need emotional support, so tend to your heart as well. As you continue to build your relationship with Dogwood, envision your body and soul unwinding and coming together in a unified state of grace.

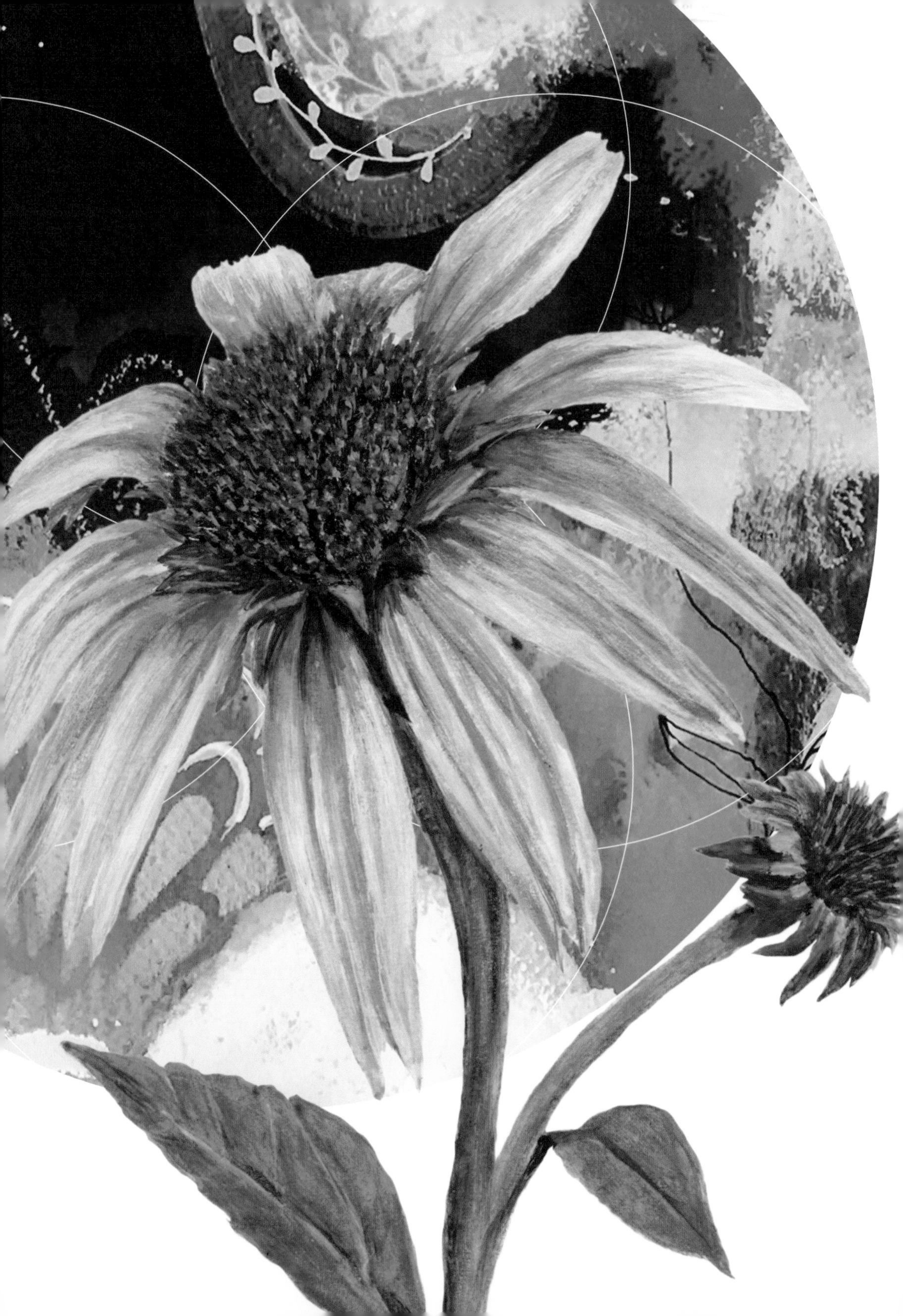

Echinacea

ECHINACEA FLOWER ESSENCE WILL ASSIST YOU WITH:

- Healing severe trauma
- Uncovering your sense of self
- Awakening the soul

Invocation

Sit outside in a garden, a park, or your yard. Take this flower essence with you and lie down or sit comfortably. After taking it, feel your connection to the earth and the simplicity that brings. Be aware of yourself and that you are held here. May your healing journey be full of grace.

An abundant herbaceous plant also known as Purple Coneflower, this hardy pollinator is native to much of North America. Echinacea flower essence is for those who have been negatively affected by the traumas of modern-day living, in which a disconnection from the earth, community, and family may take place. A lack of deep contentment within can become rampant the more disconnected we become from our true selves. Further, when one experiences violence or other forms of trauma, a more severe disconnect from the inherently joyful nature of the soul can take place. Echinacea helps restore that connection and inspire integration of the conscious and subconscious mind. After taking this essence, along with other modalities of support, a person's inner life may feel more peace and affinity, as well as more connectedness to life itself.

Evening Primrose

EVENING PRIMROSE FLOWER ESSENCE WILL ASSIST YOU WITH:

- Mending feelings of rejection
- Healing avoidant attachment in relationships
- Inspiring emotionally secure bonds

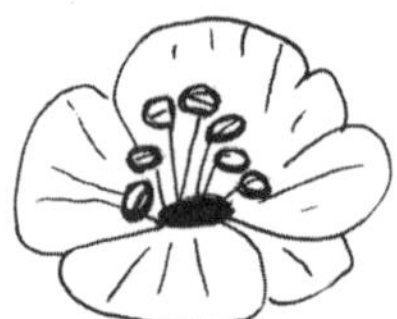

Invocation

Wrap a warm blanket around you, light a candle, and imbibe this flower essence. Visualize how you have your own mother within, and she is there for you. Breathe deep into your heart and sacral chakra (just below the belly). Feel the warmth that it brings. Trust that you can slowly open up to forming safe emotional bonds in relationships.

A fast-growing perennial herb that is native to western parts of the United States and Baja, Mexico, this herb with yellow flowers is also used medicinally. Evening Primrose flower essence can help assuage painful repressed emotions that start as early as in the womb. Our in-utero and early infant experiences are highly influential for emotional patterning later in life. If we feel at all rejected by our mother, we can form avoidant attachment styles in which we are afraid to love. Evening Primrose assists us in warming up to emotional connections that are fulfilling and nourishing for the heart. Fears of rejection may lessen, as may fears of becoming a parent or having children. An integration of repressed emotions can come back to the soul after taking this essence, thus motivating us to become more aware of our own patterns so that we can form healthy, secure bonds with others and within ourselves.

Mariposa Lily

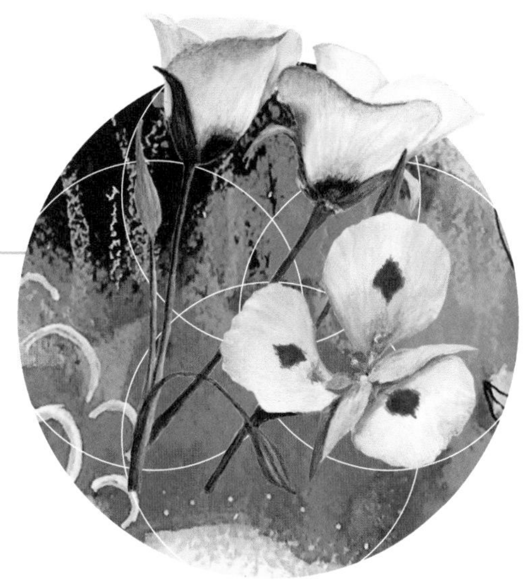

MARIPOSA LILY FLOWER ESSENCE WILL ASSIST YOU WITH:

- Healing issues of abandonment
- Heartening the inner child
- Integrating the Divine Mother within

Invocation

Sit under a large tree, such as a live oak, with a robust trunk that provides ample shade. Take Mariposa Lily flower essence and feel how Mother Earth and this tree are in support of you, holding you. Allow the internal mothering or nurturing aspect of yourself to awaken. Feel how you are safely loved by the wisdom of nature in this moment.

A part of the lily family, this perennial herb—with white petals, a yellow center, and purple spots—is native to the western United States. Mariposa Lily flower essence is all about how much maternal love and care we received as children. Many children have not received the attention and nourishment they need, which can be due to a variety of circumstances. This flower essence is about healing that much-needed bond. It inspires feelings of warmth and sustenance from within one's own heart and being. The inner child that resides within all of us can feel held by the light of the Universal Mother, the Divine Mother that sustains us all. It is valuable to spend time in nature for this healing to more effectively take place, so that you can sense a feeling of connection with Gaia, Pachamama, or Mother Earth. The gift of Mariposa Lily is that it inspires that warm, loving presence within and allows fear of giving this type of love to others to lessen.

Self-Heal

SELF-HEAL FLOWER ESSENCE WILL ASSIST YOU WITH:

- Motivation to seek healing
- Taking responsibility for your well-being
- Stirring a vitality and wellness within

Invocation

Any time you feel your energy going south or out of center, or when you start to feel ill, take the Self-Heal flower essence. It may be helpful to carry it in your purse or have it easily accessible. This handy essence is an inspiration for us to continue on the path of integration of body, mind, and heart.

An edible herbaceous plant with a rich folkloric history, this sweet little flower is found throughout Asia, Europe, and North America. Self-Heal flower essence is a fundamental energetic healer for those seeking generalized well-being and harmony. What is most valuable about this essence is that it inspires us to take responsibility for our own healing journey, for without that personal motivation, not much transformation can take place. Teachers, therapists, and other healers may also find this essence appropriate for their own self-care. No matter what the challenge is, be it physical, mental, emotional, or spiritual, this essence can help. It alleviates stagnation or blockage within to allow restoring energies to flow so that wholeness and harmony can be experienced. Know that joy is your inherent birthright. Allow Self-Heal to be an ally on your journey.

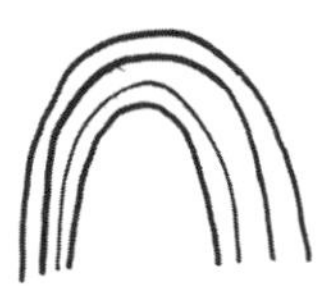

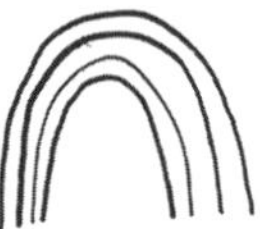

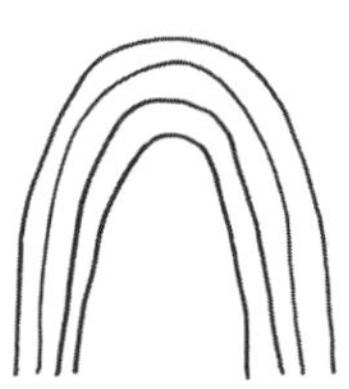

Star of Bethlehem

STAR OF BETHLEHEM FLOWER ESSENCE WILL ASSIST YOU WITH:

- Healing trauma or shock
- Feeling soothed and reassured
- Inspiring a sense of divinity

Invocation

Take Star of Bethlehem essence and find a comfortable, quiet place in your home to sit. Breathe deeply into wherever you feel stagnation, tension, or even feelings of hurt. Visualize how this gentle yet restorative healer is there to assist in your integration.

Native to most of Europe and northwestern Africa, this bulbous flowering plant has star-shaped white petals. Star of Bethlehem calms and soothes the nervous system from deep within and helps alleviate the effects of trauma. Through finding practices that nourish the body-mind-spirit connection, a person can transform and heal from past challenges more gracefully, instead of turning to addictive habits that temporarily numb feelings but can cause much more harm later. Along with seeking professional help, this essence is an important ally. Its energetic properties work with anxiety, stress, or any other nervous system dysfunction. Star of Bethlehem is a wonderful soothing formula that can bring about feelings of connection to the divine source within.

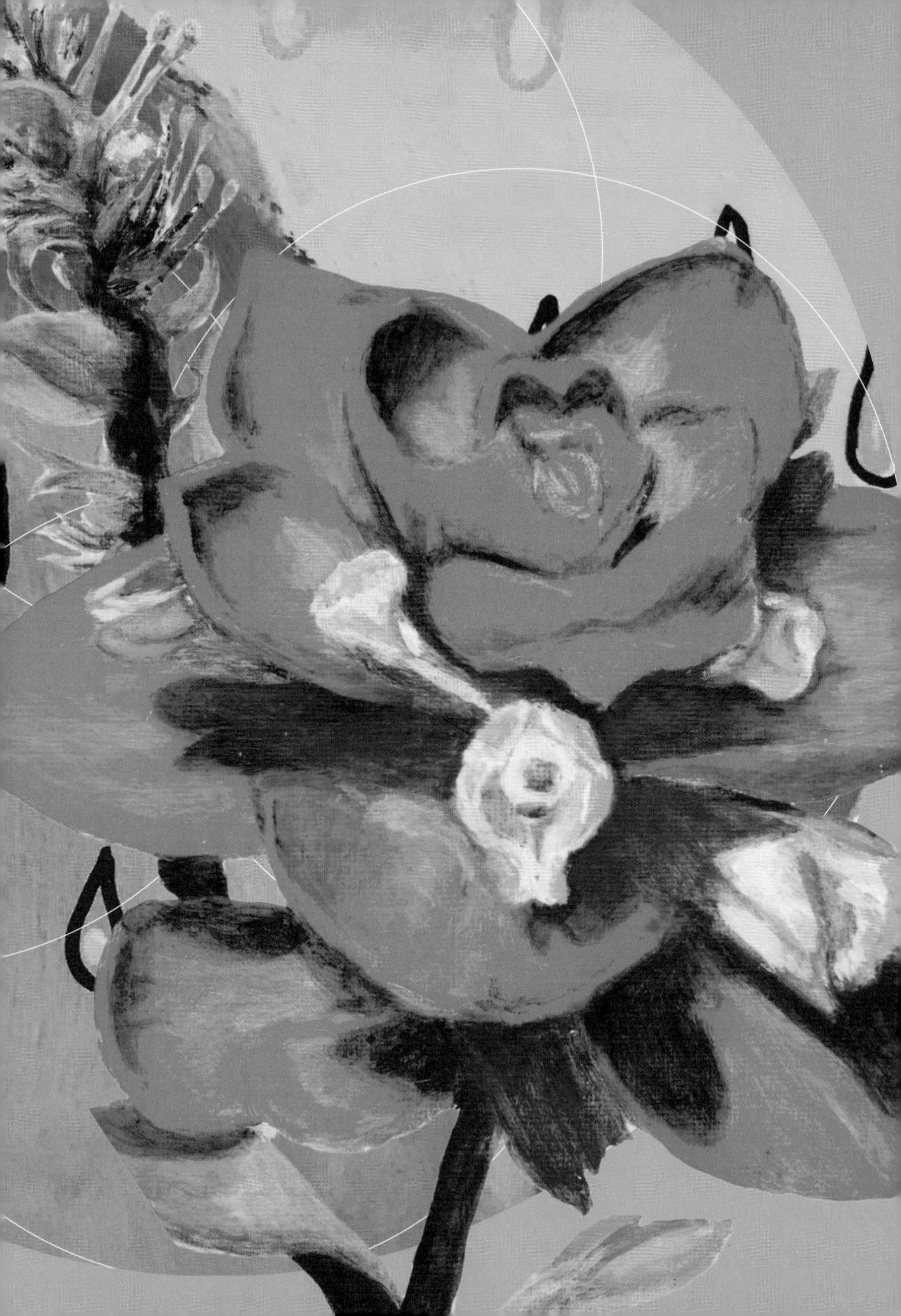

12 Flower Essences for Inspiration

"

When we love, we always strive to become better than we are. When we strive to become better than we are, everything around us becomes better too.

— Paulo Coelho

The word *inspiration* can be overused at times, so what does it truly mean to be inspired? Inspiration is akin to the art of receiving or drawing from the things around us to allow our soul to become aflame with an idea, then taking action to communicate it. To live an inspired life is to live a whole life. Inspiration does not come cheap, however. It takes discipline to continually show up to what brings us real joy. Inspiration, in a certain way, is something we need to court to bring it closer to us. So many things can be inspirational, and it can be different for every individual. To know and be true to oneself is a means of staying inspired. For an artist to find inspiration, sometimes it's just about being in the studio and getting to work. Inspiration has a way of landing when we show up for ourselves. In the end, perhaps inspiration can touch down the most when we are truthful with ourselves, engaged, and in alignment with our purpose. When our thoughts become aligned with our actions, inspiration has the chance to come along for the ride.

Columbine

COLUMBINE FLOWER ESSENCE WILL ASSIST YOU WITH:

- Unblocking creativity
- Encouraging the ability to take risks
- Inspiring expression of yourself

Invocation

Whatever your favorite way to express yourself is (e.g., dancing, making art, singing, playing music, or cooking), take this flower essence before you do your creative work. If you have felt blocked lately, do not worry. Inspiration will come back. Slowly keep showing up, and you will find the flow again.

Decorated with ornate yellow and red-orange petals that attract a variety of pollinators, this wildflower is native to western North America and blooms from April to August. Use Columbine flower essence for creative block or the fear of taking a risk, especially in the name of artistic expression. When our energies become stagnant or shut down, we can feel bored with life or lose sight of what once made us feel alive and authentic to ourselves. Columbine assists in reawakening that divine force within us so we can feel our radiance and enough courage to tap into our creativity. Once feeling more inspired, we are less afraid to share it with the world, because we know we are being true to ourselves. Columbine works with our ability to share our gifts with the world and inspire others. We might even feel moved to make a speech or perform, revealing our inner light and the genius that comes from within. Let this powerful and ornate flower motivate you to reignite the spark of passion for yourself, thus warming others and moving them to do the same.

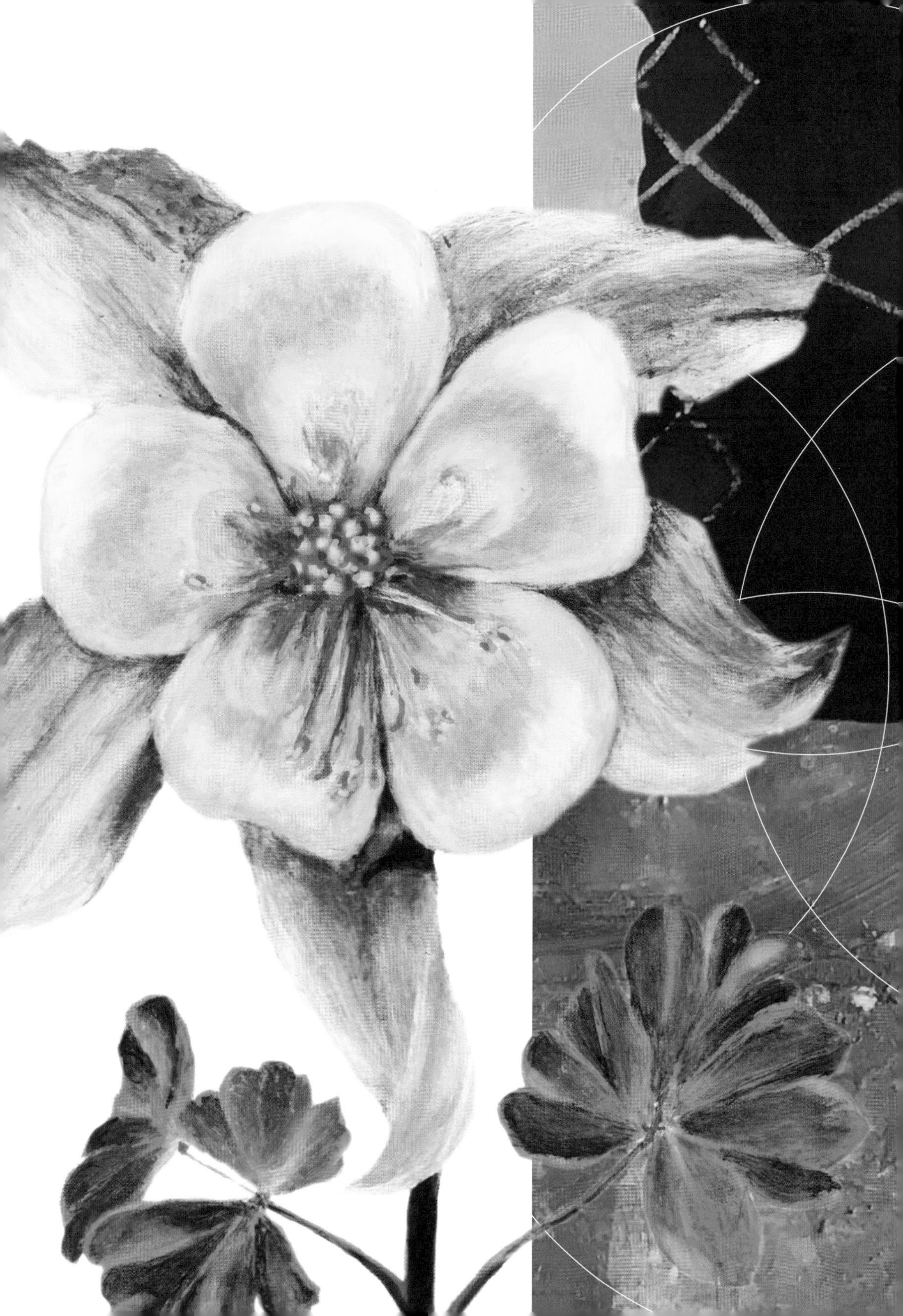

Desert Lily

DESERT LILY FLOWER ESSENCE WILL ASSIST YOU WITH:

- Finding beauty in the overwhelm of city life
- Expressing authentic creativity in modernity
- Tuning in to the power of feminine expression

Invocation

Next time you find yourself in a concrete urban environment, whether you live there or are just visiting, take this flower essence with you. Desert Lily is a balm for chaotic cities filled with technological overwhelm. When the magick of the divine feminine is needed in such environments, this essence does the trick.

Also known as the Ajo Lily, this white-petaled beauty grows in desert areas of California, Arizona, and Mexico. Desert Lily flower essence assists us with bringing feminine magick and creativity back into ourselves when in the midst of an urban culture that feels overrun by technology and capitalism. At times such environments can feel overbuilt, chaotic, and lacking in warmth and heart. Desert Lily inspires us with grace and fluidity, and it brings about the healing energy of the water element. All people, no matter their gender identity, can benefit from inspiring the divine feminine from within with this essence. Beauty, finesse, elegance, and ease are all gifts of Desert Lily. As the world and its cultural centers become more crowded and a disconnect from nature becomes apparent, this flower essence can bring about balance.

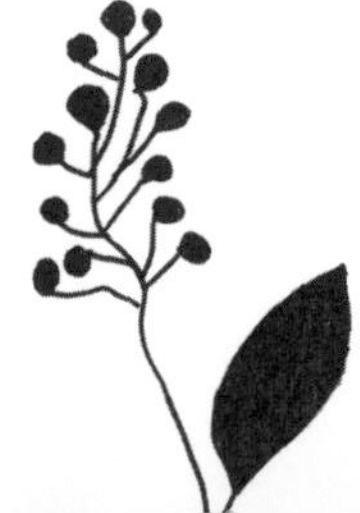

Green Rose

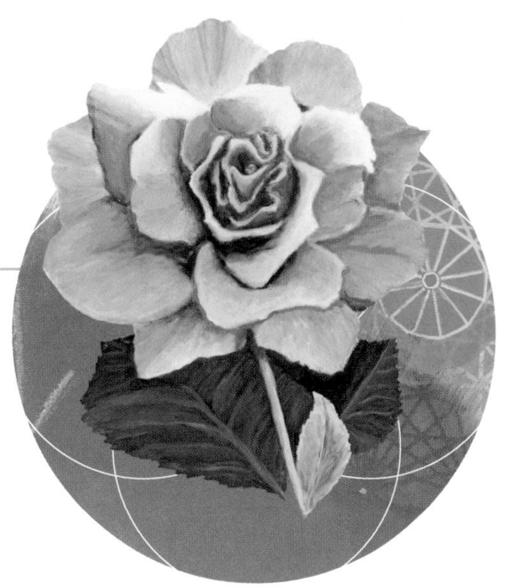

GREEN ROSE FLOWER ESSENCE WILL ASSIST YOU WITH:

- Mitigating fear and mistrust
- Letting down defensive walls within
- Inspiring transcendence and compassion

Invocation

Find a quiet place inside your home to sit and take this flower essence. After consuming it, breathe deeply and close your eyes. Visualize any barriers that you have built to protect yourself slowly dissolving. This can allow love and inspiration to flow more freely through you. Do this as a practice daily for as long as you can until you feel a shift.

A plant that is shaped like a rose but never has any petals, this perennial is thought to be a descendent of the Old Blush or China rose family. Green Rose flower essence aids in softening defensive barriers or walls within that have been built up over time. These walls served a purpose: Perhaps, for example, you have had past experiences that you needed protection from. But past traumas can live on and cause unnecessary fear and mistrust in current situations when they are no longer needed. The healing powers of the Green Rose allow those fears of being attacked to dissolve with ease and grace. This flower works its magick by transforming those feelings into compassion and inspiring real empathic connection to others. Lightness returns to the heart and the nervous system relaxes. You may begin to see humanity as something to embrace, as you realize that is exactly what you desire more of—to be warmly held with understanding by others. We give what we receive, and we are all divinely connected.

Hornbeam

HORNBEAM FLOWER ESSENCE WILL ASSIST YOU WITH:

- Overcoming fatigue and disconnection from the self
- Feeling enthusiastic about life
- Becoming more engaged with daily tasks of living

Invocation

If you can, make it a point to watch the sunrise and take this flower essence. Allow the sun's rays to fill your body with energy and notice how this essence does the same. Open yourself up to a fresh way of approaching life, one that motivates you to live true.

Native to warm climates throughout Europe and western Asia, this deciduous tree, also known as Yoke Elm, can grow up to 80 feet (24.4 m) tall. Hornbeam flower essence assists us when the daily grind of life feels draining and weariness sets in. It reawakens that enthusiasm for living—the one you have when your heart leads and feels nourished even by the most routine tasks. Hornbeam inspires the soul to feel connection to its work, and it reignites the physical form with a new vitality. A fresh perspective sets in: It is up to one's attitude and ability to make change for the better. If you have been in a rut, in which work and monotonous tasks have gotten the better of you, Hornbeam is the essence to recapture your joy in work-oriented endeavors and soul purpose.

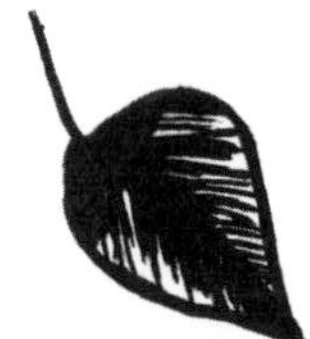

Indian Paintbrush

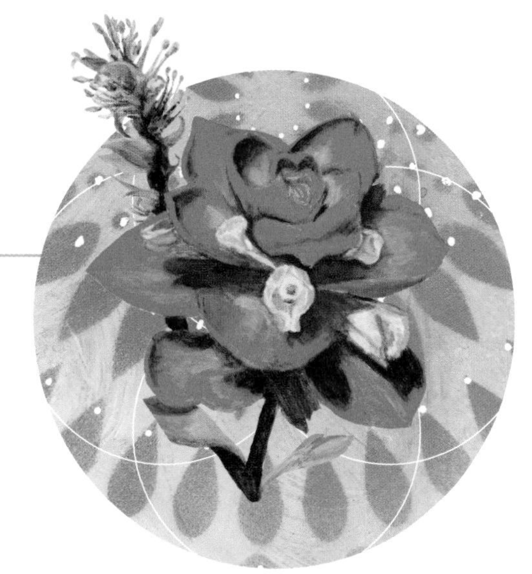

INDIAN PAINTBRUSH FLOWER ESSENCE WILL ASSIST YOU WITH:

- Unblocking creative flow
- Discovering joyful expression
- Feeling enlivened when creating

Invocation

Take Indian Paintbrush flower essence before you begin to create. Notice how your energy grounds and feels sustainable throughout your artistic process. Allow your work to deepen in meaning and intention.

Native to a wide variety of habitats in North America, this perennial herb is also known as Giant Red Indian Paintbrush. Indian Paintbrush flower essence is one of the quintessential essences for artists. It vitalizes all the energy centers, with a focus on helping artists stay grounded and balanced as they work. This helps creative souls, who are usually highly in tune and sensitive to energies anyway, to feel nourished and sustained when producing. It also inspires a bit of magick or depth to their expression or whatever they are creating. After taking this essence, an artist may find a new inspiration, one that has more meaning and connection that resonates with intention. Indian Paintbrush flower essence is a true gift for artists no matter what their media or genre, for it bestows a sense of true alignment and vision for creative expression.

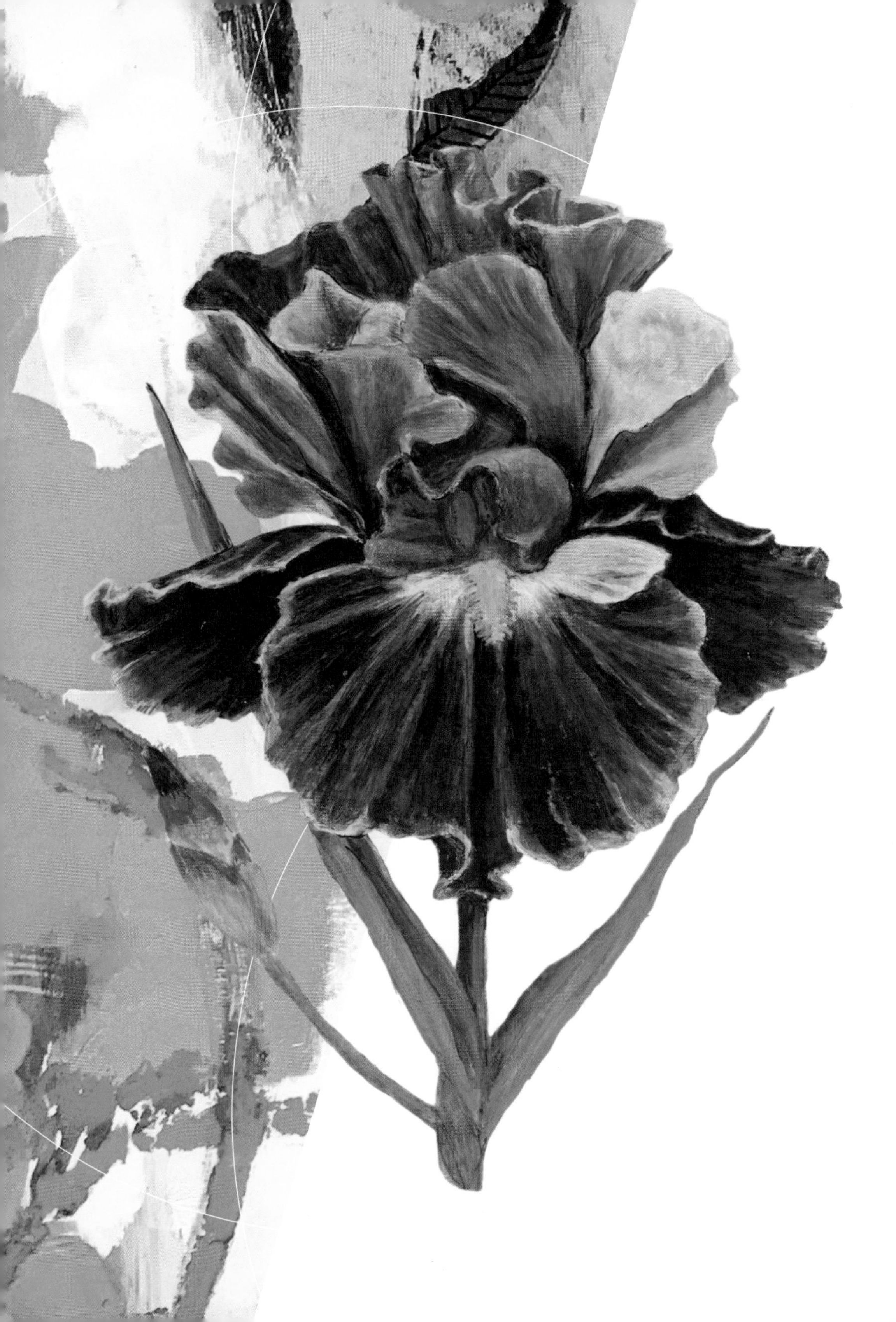

Iris

IRIS FLOWER ESSENCE WILL ASSIST YOU WITH:

- Uplifting energy for creative work
- Transforming dullness into revelation
- Bestowing radiance and inspired vision

Invocation

Before you begin your next painting, dance, song, or creative project, take this powerful essence. Iris is a flower essence for all artists. It entrusts a rich depth to your work and manifests higher vision. See how your work transforms into pure radiance after you take this essence.

A common wildflower found throughout the United States, Iris blooms from April to June with stately purple-blue petals. Iris flower essence is an incredible gift to creative people everywhere. It helps creatives who lack inspiration, insight, or expression—in other words, creatives who feel highly blocked. This essence inspires you not only to get back into the studio or onto the stage, but also to receive profound vision and resonance with other luminous realms when creating. A soul can become aflame with sharing its mystery and meaning and thus transferring itself into expression. If you want to create again, or you're seeking new ways of expressing yourself in whatever media or genre, please give Iris an opportunity to work its magick on you. Your creative juices may become radiant, iridescent, and enlivened by taking this essence. Be sure to express gratitude to Iris when this newfound inspiration lands.

Wild Oat

WILD OAT FLOWER ESSENCE WILL ASSIST YOU WITH:

- Finding direction in life
- Implementing focus and commitment
- Discovering true calling and purpose

Invocation

Take this flower essence and grab a journal in which to write. After Wild Oat starts to work its magick, begin a freewrite on your dreams in life. Write about what lights you up most inside when you think about your passions and just how you can turn them into vocations. As the weeks progress, make lists and journal some more, until you become clear on defining your calling in life.

One member of a large genus of grasses native to many temperate regions around the world, Wild Oat is a part of the cool-season lineage. This flower essence is pivotal for our modern-day culture, in which we often work as a means to get by, for monetary purposes rather than for tapping into our true calling and seeking a vocation that serves our soul. If you feel chronically bored or lackluster about your work, or you have no clear direction as to how best to serve and express your gifts, then Wild Oat can benefit you. This essence turns on your inner calling and vision for a soul path and its work, one that reflects and aligns with your true values. Once there is recognition of your full potential, inspired action can spark within, and you will experience the love and discipline you need to fulfill those dreams. Let Wild Oat spark that fire within you, so that you may go after and face your goals head-on with passion and clarity.

Wild Rose

WILD ROSE FLOWER ESSENCE WILL ASSIST YOU WITH:

- Restoring hope
- Inspiring wellness and vitality
- Feeling joyful again

Invocation

Create a healing space for yourself, one in which you can put on your favorite music, light candles, or do whatever will make you feel a little lift. Take this flower essence and allow yourself to feel all the feelings. Don't grasp or try to control them, but hold yourself. You may wish to invite a few close friends to hold you in this healing. Please also seek out help for yourself during this time. You will overcome.

A part of the rose or Rosaceae family that's native to Europe, northwest Africa, and western Asia, this climbing deciduous shrub blooms pink and white petals. Wild Rose flower essence aids in addressing lack of motivation and feelings of despair. Such hopelessness can also manifest in the physical form, where illness can take root and there is a chronic lethargy or feeling like the body's reserves are deeply depleted. Wild Rose inspires an inner well to begin to bubble again willfully and with more faith. By taking this flower essence, you may begin to feel a restoration in your heart, thus encouraging you to have more intrigue and interest in life. A connection to the whole body and its subtle layers may also take place, giving you vitality that was once lost. Once the body feels more able, the mind and heart follow suit, bringing about a joyful attitude toward life and living. Let Wild Rose help you feel how life is a beloved opportunity for growth, connection, and visceral experience.

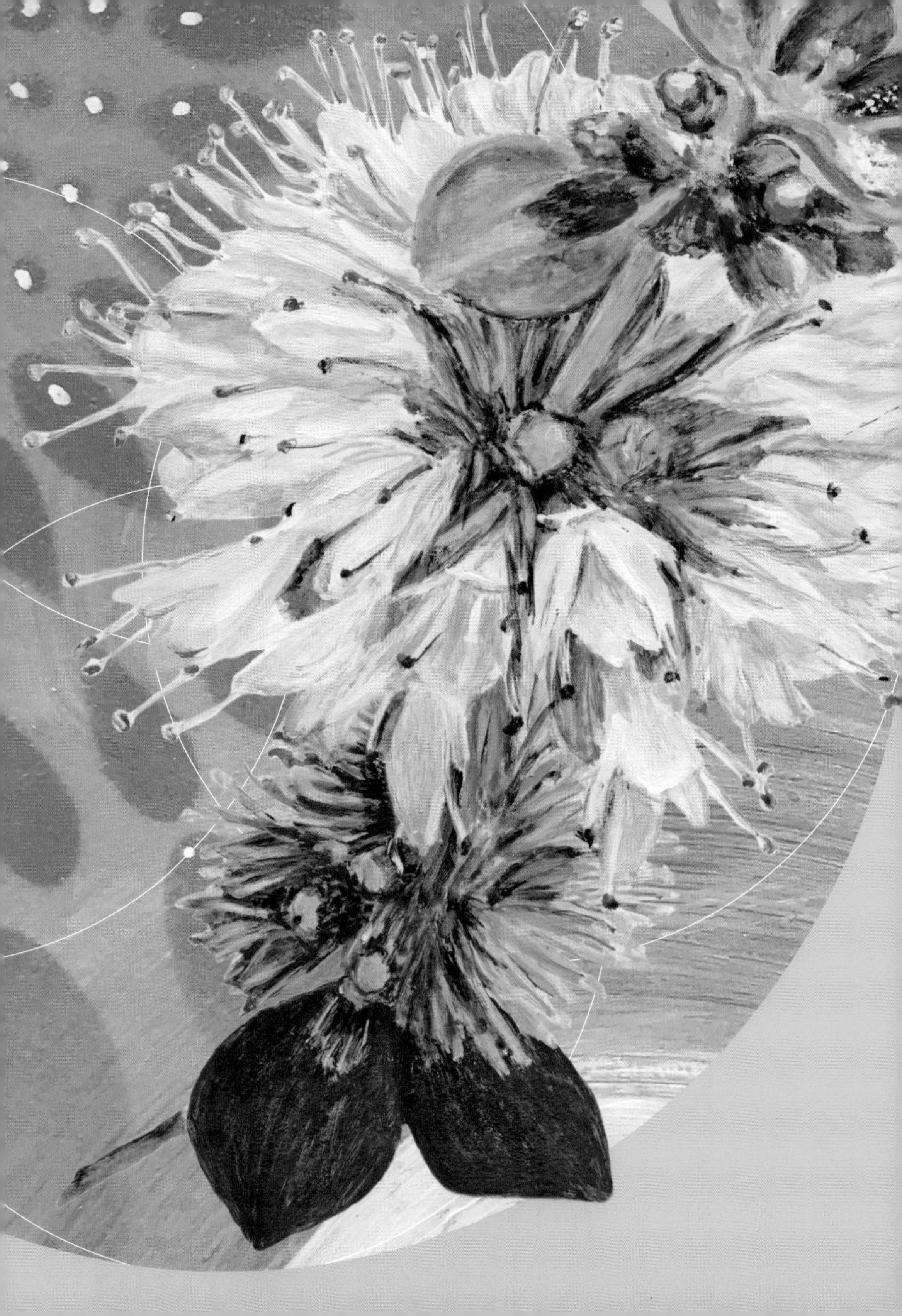

13 Flower Essences for Self-Esteem

"

You yourself, as much as anybody in the entire universe, deserve your love and affection.

—Sharon Salzberg

Having a healthy self-esteem is an integral part of living a fulfilled life. But what exactly is a healthy self-esteem? Perhaps it is feeling at home in oneself, having belief in and understanding one's value intrinsically. It also can mean seeing yourself clearly and feeling a sense of belonging and connection here on earth. Self-esteem is something we have to care for, work at, discover, and uncover. Loving oneself can be, paradoxically, both easy and difficult. A path of valuable self-worth may start with forgiveness—forgiveness toward others and toward yourself. When we forgive, we give ourselves a gift of liberation and happiness. Healthy self-esteem means knowing how to receive such gifts easily and with understanding.

California Peony

CALIFORNIA PEONY FLOWER ESSENCE WILL ASSIST YOU WITH:

- Freeing up manifestation abilities
- Strengthening chi and vitality
- Enhancing magnetism and charisma

Invocation

Take this flower essence and begin to shake, shimmy, move, and allow the vital forces from the ground to move up through your body. Yell, sing, and release whatever you need to from a primal, authentic place deep inside you. Say this out loud to yourself: "I am here, I am alive, I am beautiful, and I am worthy." That's California Peony working its magick on you.

Native to southwestern California and Baja, Mexico, this deciduous summer plant, also known as Wild Peony, grows on hillsides and in coastal regions. California Peony flower essence works on energies that are more passive or overly yin in nature. This can affect self-esteem in a variety of ways, from underproducing in life to having a repressed sex drive, one where the sensual part of oneself is cut off. If you have difficulty with feeling empowered and making enough money to sustain yourself, this flower essence is an opportune healer. The alchemy of the California Peony is that it cultivates magnetic inner vitality and touches into the sacral chakra. A thriving flow of sexuality is restored and ignited. Your disposition can shift from insecure to radiant and strong. Grant California Peony's gifts in your life by celebrating all that you are, wholly, wildly, and with luminosity.

Elm

ELM FLOWER ESSENCE WILL ASSIST YOU WITH:

- Restoring confidence
- Finding calm despite many duties
- Feeling fulfilled when doing acts of service

Invocation

Before you begin your day, take Elm flower essence and commit to doing random acts of kindness. Try doing this as often as you can. See how it makes you feel. Even with a full plate, acts of service can be beautifully rewarding.

Native to varying parts of the Eurasian continent, the Elm tree blooms in spring with reddish-brown to purple flowers and can grow up to almost 100 feet (30.5 m) in height. Elm flower essence is instrumental when dealing with overwhelm and fatigue toward life's daily tasks and responsibilities. This can be because of self-doubt or lack of motivation toward work and other responsibilities. When this type of despondency sets in, Elm can ignite self-worth and courage to get the job done. This essence takes it a step further, too: It inspires an enthusiastic attitude toward helping others from a place of joy along with living out your soul purpose. Elm can inspire you to take a guiding role, one in which you can lead or teach others to listen to their calling and intuition. In sum, this potent essence quiets despondency and sparks confidence and authenticity toward your vocations and passions in this world.

Fawn Lily

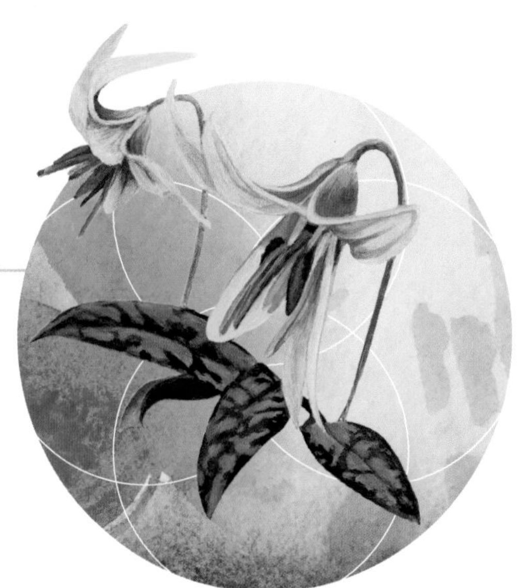

FAWN LILY FLOWER ESSENCE WILL ASSIST YOU WITH:

- Building strength and desire for connection
- Allowing your gifts to be seen
- Becoming more involved in communities

Invocation

Take Fawn Lily flower essence and head out for some time in town or for a group activity. Feel yourself open to connection with others, realizing you have many gifts to share. Notice how valuable it is to be involved in community. How can you show up more, allow yourself to be seen, and share your many gifts with others? The world needs you; it's time to find that balance between introversion and extroversion.

Also known as the Purple Fawn Lily, this mountain wildflower, with its purple and yellow base petals, can reach up to 8 inches (20 cm) tall and is native to California. Fawn Lily flower essence is for highly sensitive individuals who are most comfortable in spiritual practice and contemplation. It can be difficult for them to cope with and be a part of modern life. Because these souls are so adept with meditation and other internal methods of connection, their ability to connect with others and interact in the world can run dry. This leads to an imbalance within. The drawback of isolation is the inability to share one's gifts in community. Fawn Lily flower essence is suggested for a more holistic integration. This healer will inspire these individuals to become healers themselves, allowing their gifts to be seen. If any of the above description fits you, allow Fawn Lily to spark that desire for the benefits of welcoming more human connection into your life. The world desires your light.

Goldenrod

GOLDENROD FLOWER ESSENCE WILL ASSIST YOU WITH:

- Strengthening your sense of sovereignty
- Expressing yourself authentically
- Feeling whole and connected in group settings

Invocation

Go into a large group setting or social event and take Goldenrod flower essence. Allow yourself to feel your individuality and trust it. Express who you are without worrying about group mentality. Trust your uniqueness.

Native to western areas of the United States, this perennial herb, which is also used medicinally, has golden yellow flowers that can grow up to 5 feet (1.5 m) tall. Goldenrod flower essence is ideal for those who tend to get morphed into a group or community mind-set and lose their sense of self. This flower essence is also beneficial for codependency or enabling patterns in relationships. If you tend to be overly influenced by others and have a hard time deciding what you actually feel and truly want to express, this flower essence can be of service to you. Goldenrod can embolden you to find your connection to source and authenticity, even when in group settings. This potent flower essence allows you to integrate a sense of true self when relating to others, freeing up the ties that bind you, which may have developed because of challenging experiences in your early childhood development. It is a pertinent healer for self-esteem because it inspires the genuine self to shine through, despite familial or community pressures.

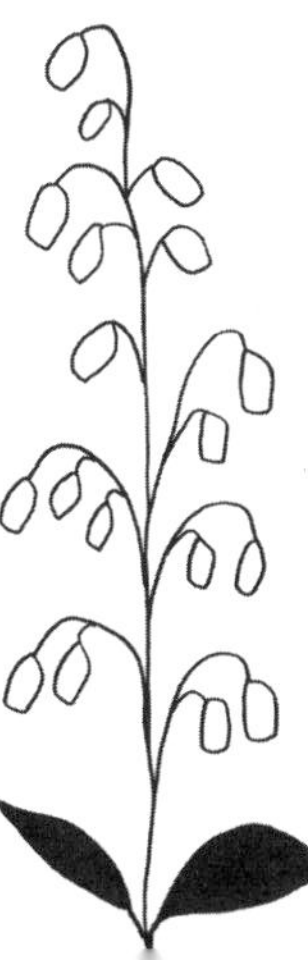

Larkspur

LARKSPUR FLOWER ESSENCE WILL ASSIST YOU WITH:

- Balancing a self-aggrandized ego
- Leading from a place of joy
- Inspiring service-oriented work

Invocation

Next time you prepare yourself to be with a group of people or in a leadership role, take this flower essence beforehand. Set an intention to lead from your heart and not your head. See how your interactions with others change. How did this make you feel? Allow this transformation to take place when surrounding yourself with others.

This wildflower comes in a variety of colors and is native across North America. Larkspur flower essence is essential when your ego has become too self-important and controlling. This can be caused by self-esteem issues, which may have developed much earlier due to your upbringing or lack of attention to you. The ego's job is to protect and strategize, so it wants positions of power. Larkspur helps remedy this and bring about heart-based leadership. This can be quite liberating because it inspires authenticity, joy, and dedication to serving others. It assists in breaking the chains of ego-driven personality. In essence, Larkspur aligns you with your whole being and connection to source, thus bringing about more meaningful relationships and connections. This also galvanizes others to follow your leadership willingly and with trust.

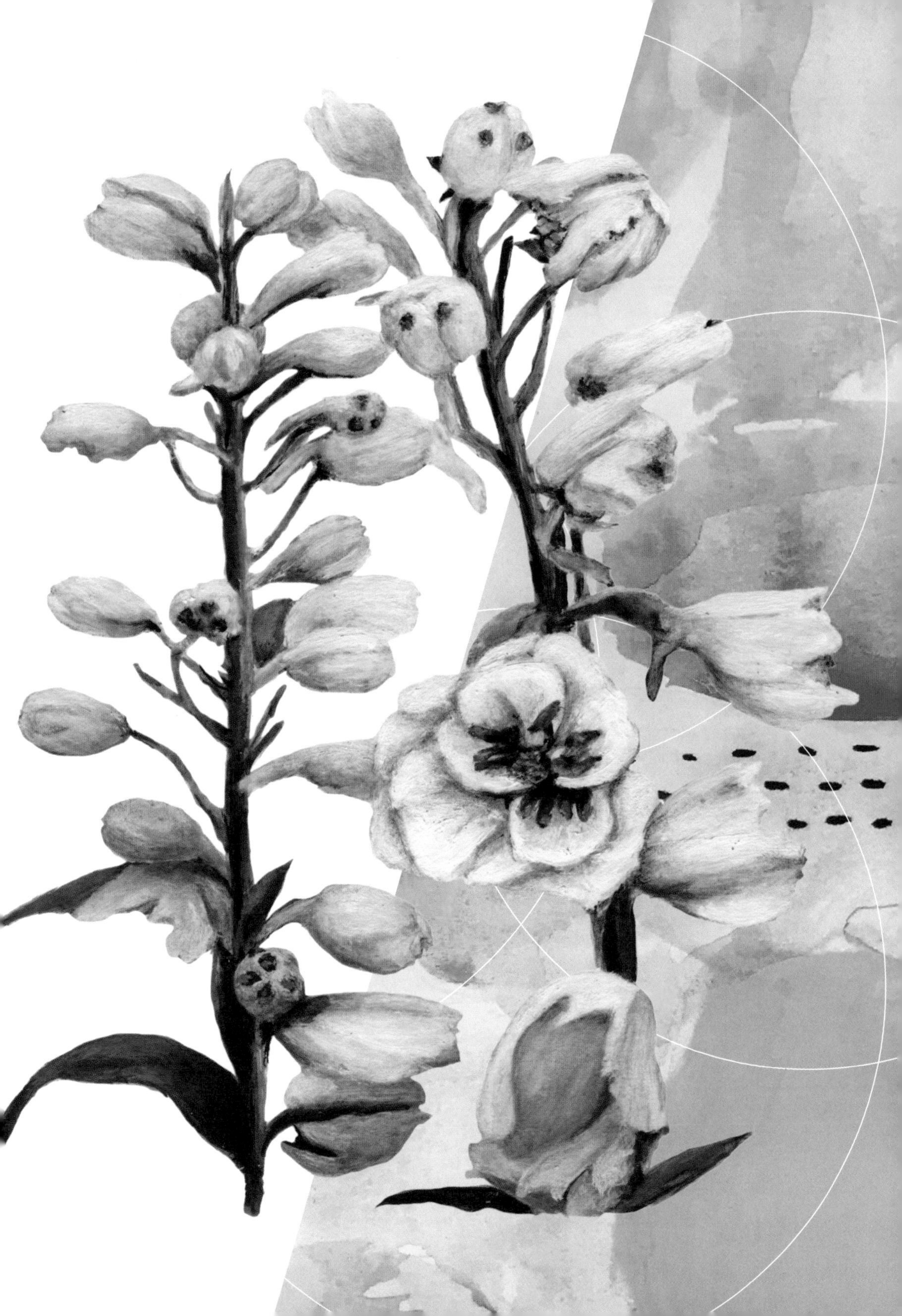

Mallow

MALLOW FLOWER ESSENCE WILL ASSIST YOU WITH:

- Dissolving barriers in the heart
- Bringing about warmth from within
- Sparking openheartedness

Invocation

Take this flower essence with you when you are planning to be with others, whether romantically or in a group environment. Upon taking it, notice the warmth it can inspire in your heart. Envision your heart opening up like a lotus or rose, ready and willing to give and receive love.

Found in mountain meadow habitats, this California-native perennial herb has pink-violet petals. Mallow flower essence is fitting for those who have learned to mistrust others, especially in matters of the heart. Likely because of their past, these souls have built protective layers around themselves and have not been able to fully open up to love, connection, or a sense of belonging with friends or loved ones. Mallow assists in dissolving those walls and igniting a warmth and receptivity inside. This can bring about many gifts for those who have felt shut down for some time. True love and connection in many forms of relationships can take root. A flow of giving and receiving—which is natural to humans—can take place, thus fulfilling the abilities of the heart. If you have felt closed off to real love and connection, allow Mallow to gently open you up to this possibility and receive its blessing.

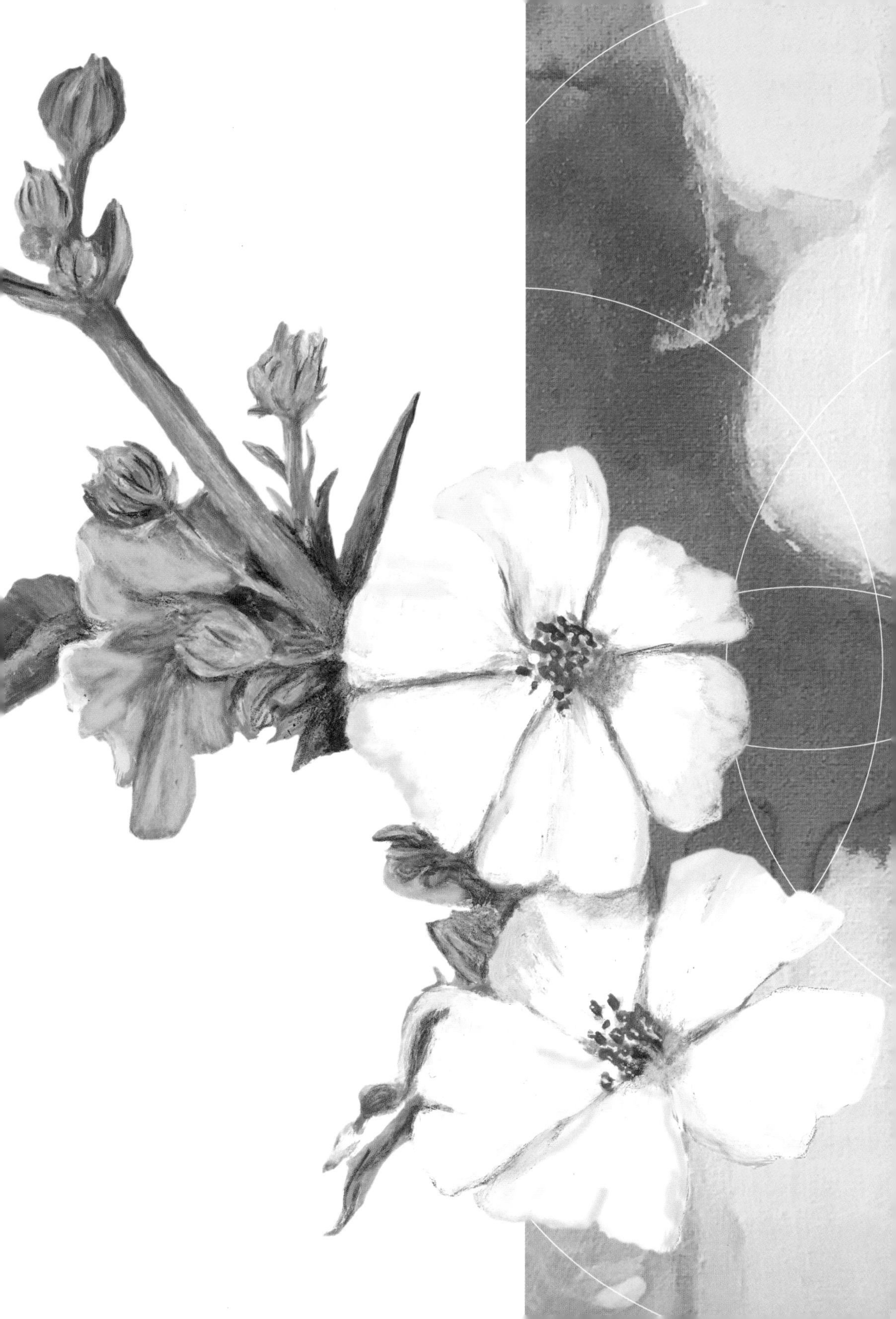

Mountain Pennyroyal

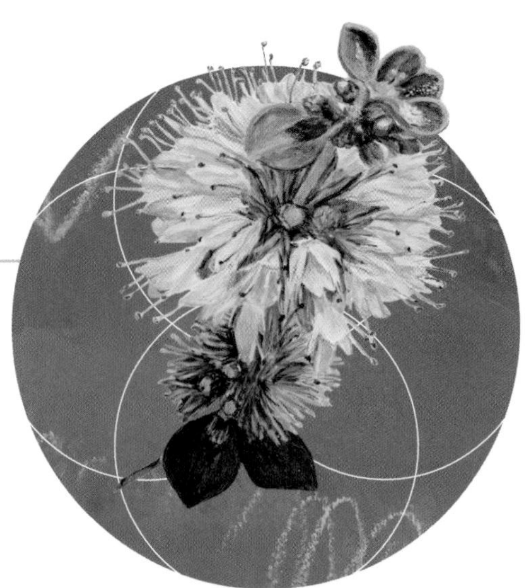

MOUNTAIN PENNYROYAL FLOWER ESSENCE WILL ASSIST YOU WITH:

- Establishing a protected field
- Inspiring positivity and clarity
- Building vitality and strength

Invocation

Before you exercise, take a hot bath, or do anything during which you plan to sweat and cleanse your body, take this flower essence. Mountain Pennyroyal is all about cleansing and strengthening your auric field. Feel the clarity this essence brings.

A member of the mint family, this sprawling perennial herb is native to western parts of the United States, especially California. Mountain Pennyroyal flower essence inspires clear perception to the mental body. It does this by cleansing negativity and psychic toxicity from the mind. Empaths and healers especially have trouble with this, because they can pick up too much energy from others around them that then gets stored in their own heads. Mountain Pennyroyal is a protective essence that strengthens one's own energy, building sovereignty and restoring optimism and integration. If you have been picking up too much on society's mental conditioning and the doubts of others, Mountain Pennyroyal may be perfect for you. Allow this essence to purge those belief systems that were never yours to begin with, so you can lead your life with expansive and clear thinking.

Prettyface

PRETTYFACE FLOWER ESSENCE WILL ASSIST YOU WITH:

- Letting go of obsession with physical appearance
- Building self-esteem in relation to physicality
- Understanding that true beauty lies within

Invocation

Take Prettyface flower essence and then go look at yourself in the mirror. Closing your eyes in front of the mirror, breathe in the energy of the essence. Then slowly open your eyes. See the light and beauty coming from within. Your true magnetism is irreplaceable. Begin to live and remember that.

Also known as Golden Star, this perennial wildflower can be found in coastal and inland forest habitats. Prettyface flower essence is incredibly apropos for the times we are living in. In this age of social media and selfies, there is high value placed on how one looks physically alongside unrealistic and competitive beauty standards. This essence helps balance out this obsessive energy and superficiality. Prettyface teaches us that true beauty lies within a human being, for that is where the radiance comes from. It is also a valuable healer for those born disfigured or with deformity, so they can come into a place of peace and acceptance of the way they look and how they see themselves. This flower essence helps one begin to understand that true beauty and luminosity only come from inside one's soul, therefore directing attention inside rather than outside.

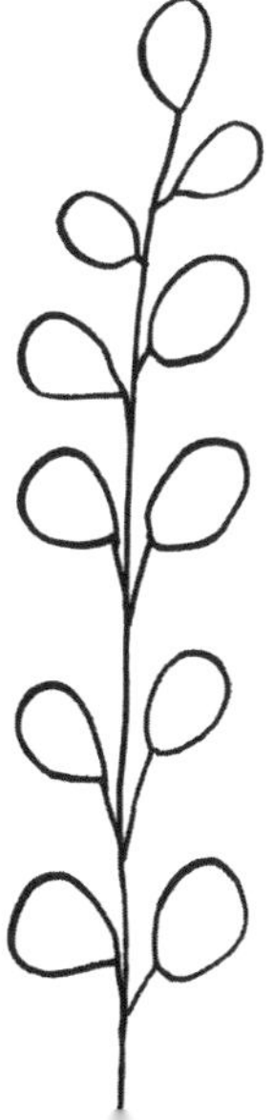

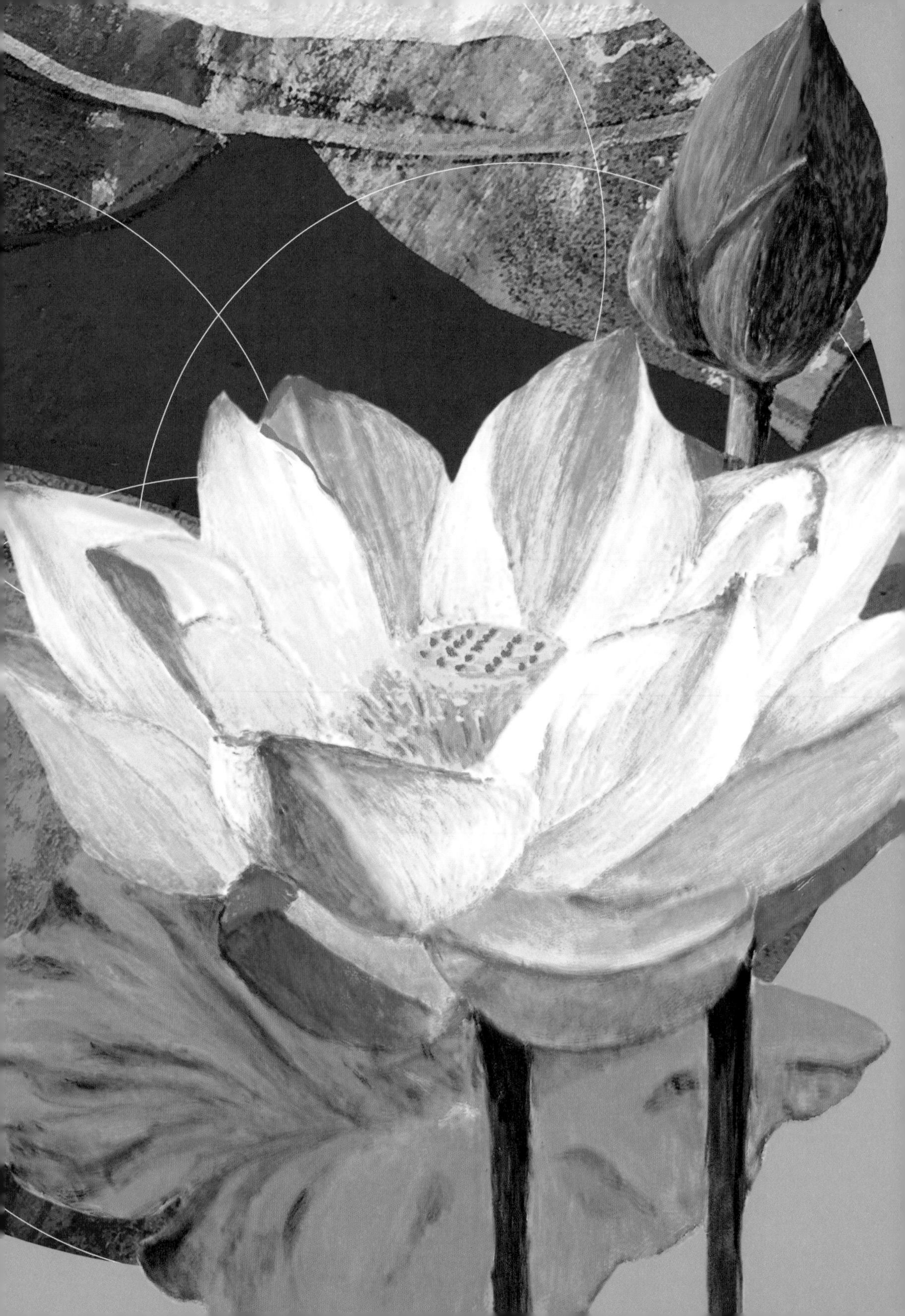

14 Flower Essences for Transformation

"

Sorrow prepares you for joy. It violently sweeps everything out of your house, so that new joy can find space to enter. It shakes the yellow leaves from the bough of your heart, so that fresh, green leaves can grow in their place. It pulls up the rotten roots, so that new roots hidden beneath have room to grow. Whatever sorrow shakes from your heart, far better things will take their place.

— Rumi

Some say that life is about the journey, not the destination. It is a process of learning, unlearning, and transformation. The soul comes here to evolve and has the gift of embodying a human form, in which learning is intense and perpetual. Transformation allows us to integrate into wholehearted living or living from a place of love. To be loved, share love, give love, and know love deeply . . . these are the gifts of having a human life. How auspicious that so many flowers can represent integration, love, and real growth. They themselves grow from the perfect balance of sun, water, and earth. Nature is a representation of the mystery—the power and magical force that is source itself. Flowers are an auspicious part of that mystery. This chapter features some flowers that can aid you on your journey of transformation.

Alpine Aster

ALPINE ASTER FLOWER ESSENCE WILL ASSIST YOU WITH:

- Letting go of materialism
- Realizing deeper states of consciousness
- Detaching from your body during death

Invocation

Take a blanket and go lie down under a big tree. Take this flower essence and feel all parts of your consciousness, beyond your body. Focus on your third eye in between your eyebrows, your heart chakra, and the rest of your body. Notice just your consciousness and begin to feel its vastness, even beyond your human form.

Native to the mountains of Europe, this ornamental perennial has purple, blue, or pink flowers. Alpine Aster flower essence gives us the gift of transcendence and deeper awakening of consciousness beyond the material and physical, or what only appears to be real. It aids in releasing materialistic bonds and gives the powerful understanding of other spiritual dimensions and realities. Alpine Aster is an opportune flower essence for meditation. It supports opening up vast, deeper layers of consciousness beyond the body. Use it if you want to experience lucid dreaming or astral travel. Alpine Aster can also help during death, allowing the transition to be smoother and more harmonious.

Cayenne

CAYENNE FLOWER ESSENCE WILL ASSIST YOU WITH:

- Releasing stagnation
- Embodying more energetic vitality and fire
- Inspiring transformation

Invocation

Take this flower essence and then move your body about rapidly. Shake, shimmy, yell, dance, sweat—get that energy moving. Cayenne is all about the transformation of backed-up energy. It is time to feel your passion for life again.

Part of the nightshade family, this woody shrub with white star flowers is best known for producing edible hot peppers, but it is also used for its medicinal herbal properties. Cayenne flower essence is for the stimulation of stagnant energies. If you have been feeling in a slump or overly lethargic lately, let this flower essence spice and shake up things for you. Or, if your energy has been damp or even cold and aloof in nature, let the fire of this potent essence spark some vitality into your being. Its healing properties call for natural transformation, but in lively and passionate ways. Cayenne can propel you forward past your own blocks, thus sparking exciting change and new possibilities. You are here to live life to the fullest with a heart ablaze with love.

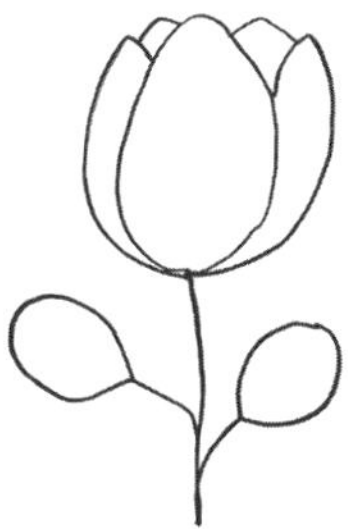

Lilac

LILAC FLOWER ESSENCE WILL ASSIST YOU WITH:

- Alleviating sadness or depression
- Calling for more connection
- Heartening real joy and meaning

Invocation

Take this flower essence and go sit in a quiet and comfortable area. Place your hand over your heart and breathe into the core of your being. Allow the warmth of your hands to bring you comfort. Feel your connection and envision yourself lifting out of this sadness. Know you are held here in love.

A large, sweet-smelling deciduous shrub that has made its way all around the world due to its attractive qualities, the Lilac is native to varying parts of Europe, and it has a rich history. Lilac flower essence provides comfort to those remembering early childhood, especially if it was difficult and is still affecting their present-day awareness—for example, if they are still experiencing feelings of abandonment and alienation. This compelling healer inspires a lift out of depressed states into a meaningful, fulfilled life. Restoration and rejuvenation of the soul may take place, causing real joy and understanding of life. Kinder and more loving memories may resurface, allowing the mind to fall into alignment with the tenderness and kind nature of the heart. Bring Lilac into your life if you could use some more healing from the past, especially early childhood, and desire to integrate into your true state of contentment once again.

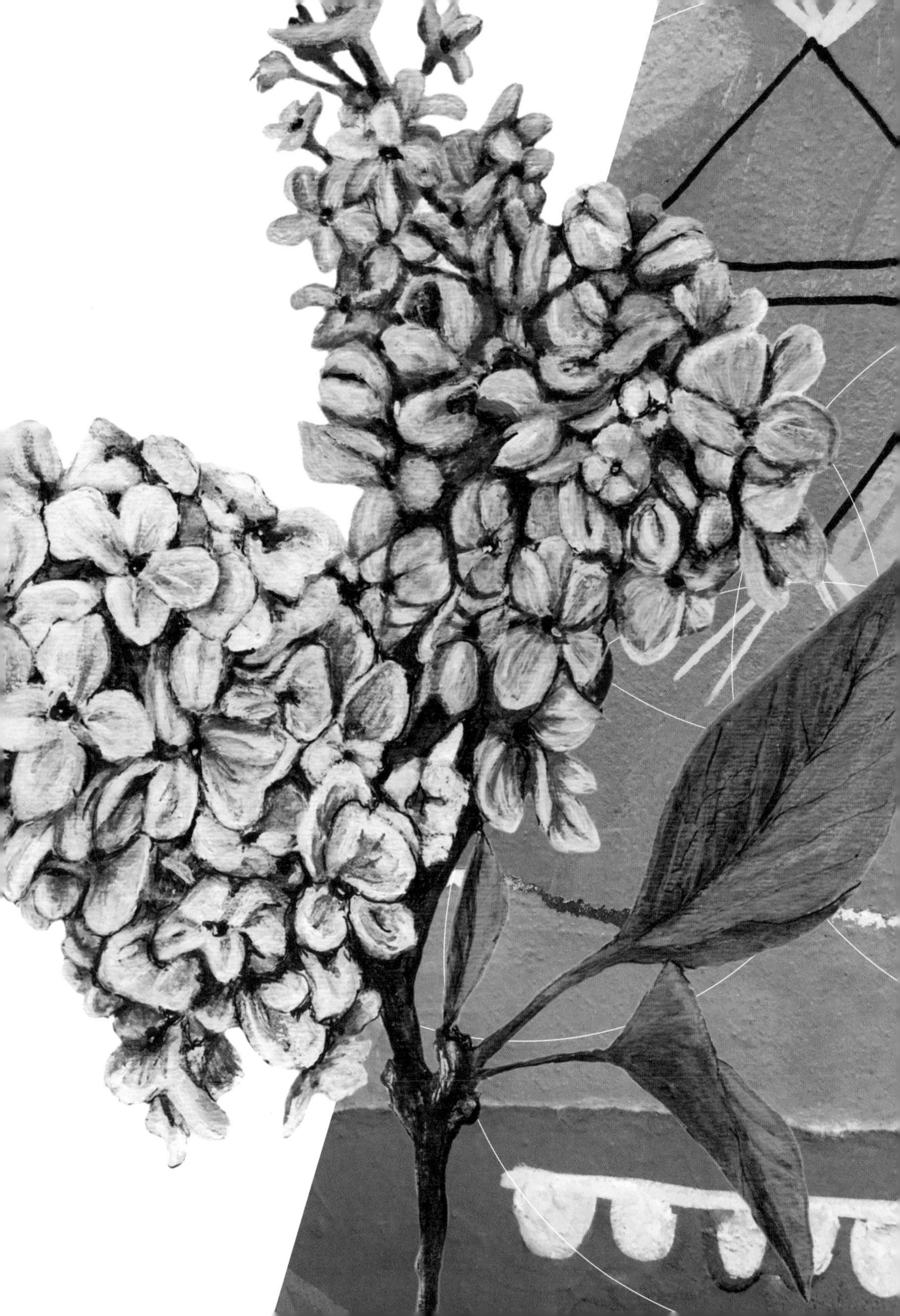

Lotus

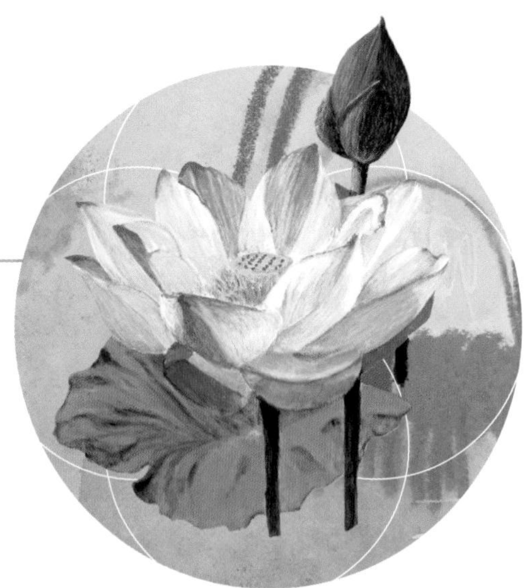

LOTUS FLOWER ESSENCE WILL ASSIST YOU WITH:

- Embodying humility
- Deepening spiritual understanding
- Encouraging service to the world

Invocation

Take this flower essence with you to a public place to observe humanity and nature. After taking it, breathe into your heart center and feel the world around you. Ask to become aligned with the real nature of things and know the truth about yourself. Ask for humility and to be shown how to be of more service to others. The asking and doing bring profound gifts of transformation.

A genus of aquatic plants, these divine flowers have a wide history of sacred meaning in Eastern regions, and they are used in traditional Chinese medicine. Lotus flower essence helps you understand what it means to be humble and how that is the pathway to real enlightenment. If you are drawn to a more spiritual way of life through study, your ego can become inflated. Lotus brings about balance and a more inclusive spiritual self, one that expands beyond focusing solely on needs and desire. From this understanding, liberation can take place, and you can be inspired to give back more to the world, for all reality is interwoven and innately connected. In other words, there are no others; we are all held in the vast network of life.

Lupine

LUPINE FLOWER ESSENCE WILL ASSIST YOU WITH:

- Overcoming greed and self-centeredness
- Inspiring an ability to serve
- Belonging to a community

Invocation

Take Lupine flower essence with you next time you walk downtown or into an urban environment where you may see others in need. Notice what judgments or perceptions shift within you. How did it make you feel? Does it inspire you to reach out and serve the whole of humanity more? Let Lupine transform your sense of self into a sense of all.

Native to western parts of the United States and British Columbia, this perennial herb bears many purple to white flowers vertically, sometimes up to 12 inches (30 cm) in height. Lupine flower essence is fitting for those who are stuck in overidentification with the self and its needs. Needs can turn into greed when you don't see the entire connection to humanity, that we are all a part of one human family. This flower essence helps transform selfishness into service, so you will feel a sense of belonging and connection to a greater good and calling. This is a gift for the soul—one that liberates the ego out of center staging. If you have found yourself feeling more self-interested and have not helped others in some time, consider taking Lupine to bring about more inner contentment and fulfillment. You will find this to be a path of liberation, out of the suffering of separation and "what's mine is mine" mentality.

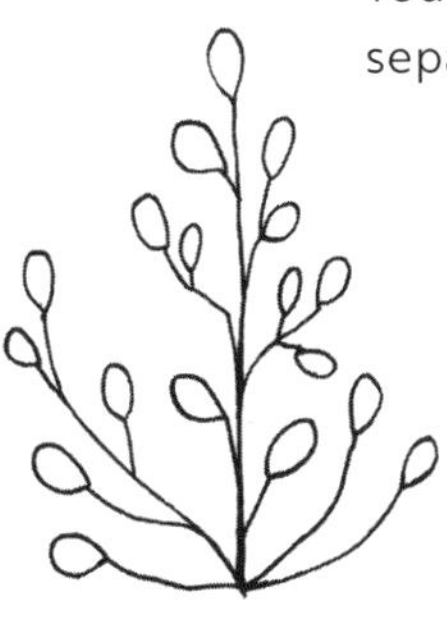

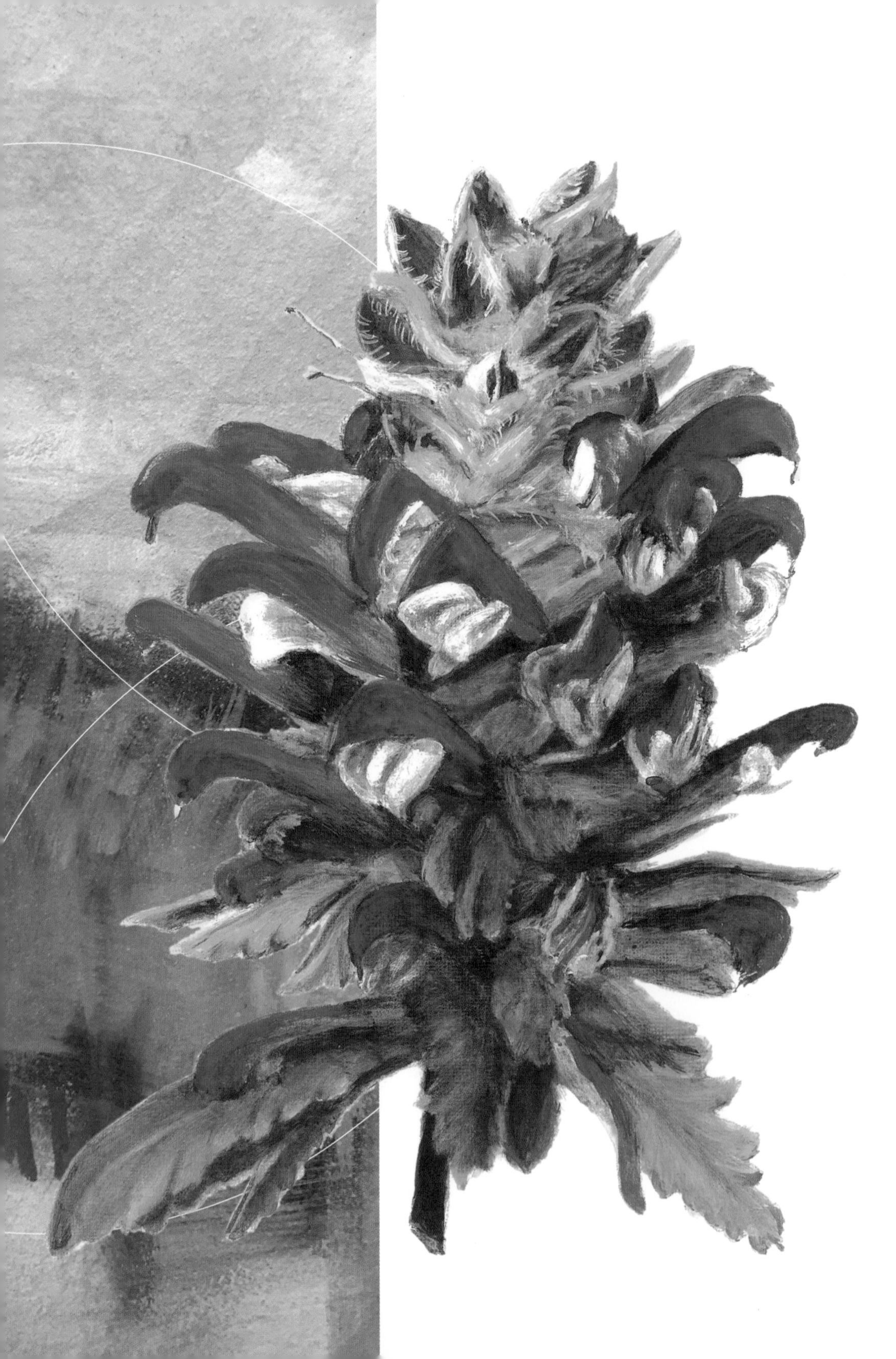

Pedicularis

PEDICULARIS FLOWER ESSENCE WILL ASSIST YOU WITH:

- Overidentifying with watery emotions
- Deepening perseverance for the soul
- Integrating soul memory and insight

Invocation

Take this flower essence when you feel your emotions rising and breathe deeply into your core. Visualize the water element within calming and settling down all the way into your feet. Ground here and breathe into the earth. Feel how you are supported.

This erect herb with ornate flowers can grow up to 32 inches (80 cm) in height; it's native to the United States and grows in wet riverbanks and high mountain ranges. Pedicularis flower essence calms and soothes an overactive emotional body, one that reacts easily and pours out tears often. This can develop in highly refined and sensitive souls for many reasons. They can find refuge and balance in calming and grounding their sensitivity so they can thrive in today's world. Pedicularis aids in bringing those emotions into balance. It turns on profound and mystical insight within so that understanding and transformation can take place. By taking this flower essence, one can become uplifted into more optimistic states of consciousness. Pedicularis grants the soul spiritual knowledge from the past and a more intimate connection with earth wisdom. If you have found yourself taken over by watery emotions lately, allow this flower essence to bestow its magick and power within you with harmony and potent insight.

Sage

SAGE FLOWER ESSENCE WILL ASSIST YOU WITH:

- Negative viewpoints toward life
- Gathering wisdom from life experience
- Seeing things from a broader perspective

Invocation

Alongside taking this flower essence, take out your journal and begin to write the story of your life and experience. Allow this to be a freewriting exercise without any censorship. Now go back and read what you wrote. What do you notice about your perception? Are certain themes popping up? Sage lets us see life from a deeper perspective and gives us a sense of purpose. Continue to write and take this essence and see how your thoughts shift.

A part of the mint family native to the Mediterranean, this perennial evergreen is often used in cooking and for its medical herbal properties. Sage flower essence is all about contemplation of one's journey and life experience. It grants the gifts of spiritual insight and wisdom by gathering and reflecting upon life's themes and patterns. By taking this essence, one can go from seeing life as a challenge, perhaps even in victim consciousness or with a pessimistic outlook, to understanding and empowerment. This happens when one draws wisdom and understanding from the events in one's life. From this newfound place, a soul can see from a vast perspective, one in which learned lessons become a part of one's being. This process calls for transformation; it shifts one into finding one's own meaning and higher purpose.

Shooting Star

SHOOTING STAR FLOWER ESSENCE WILL ASSIST YOU WITH:

- Healing feelings of alienation
- Increasing receptivity and warmth
- Feeling connected to earth and humanity

Invocation

Go outside and take Shooting Star essence. Sit in a comfortable place and notice how the trees dance in the wind and the leaves shimmer. Sense how you are an integral part of things, connected to the cosmos, the earth, and all humanity. Because you are here, you matter very much.

Native to western North America, this flowering plant is a summer deciduous, with petals ranging from violet to pink to white. Shooting Star flower essence is a potent healer if you have been feeling disconnected, isolated, or alienated from Earth and other humans. This can come from birth trauma or early childhood experiences, and it brings about the feeling that you do not belong here on this planet. This flower essence transforms those feelings into a belief that you do belong because you have been given a human body. It inspires resonance and warmth toward Earth and her wisdom, along with a feeling of connection to greater humanity. A greater awareness can sink in, one that connects to cosmic consciousness and fills the soul with love and kinship. You may realize that Earth is indeed home and that this is indeed the right time to be alive and to grow.

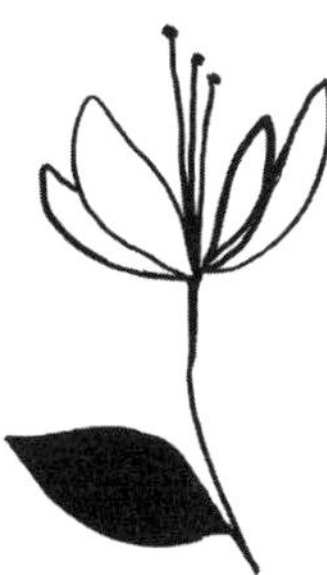

Snapdragon

SNAPDRAGON FLOWER ESSENCE WILL ASSIST YOU WITH:

- Cooling verbal frustration and anger
- Inspiring clear and balanced communication
- Harmonizing fiery energy

Invocation

Take this flower essence with you to a body of water and go swimming if you can. Or, if you dare, take a cold shower after consuming it! Snapdragon aids in cooling fiery tempers, especially when expressed verbally. Use this essence if you've been running hot lately.

An herbaceous perennial plant that is native to the Mediterranean, this stately flower is used as an ornamental in gardens. Snapdragon flower essence calms a hostile disposition, especially one that gets verbally aggressive and angry. A person who would benefit from taking this essence can have repressed or tense emotions stuck inside, and they express themselves in reactionary states. Snapdragon assists in balancing out this energy into one that is vital and lively, inspiring passion rather than emotional damage. Communication flows more with ease and grace. It may also mean the return of a healthy libido—one that expresses the need for connection through love and attraction, rather than fires that burn down relationships. If you have found yourself "snapping" at others lately and maybe even feel a little too aggravated with life, allow this flower essence to transform those feelings into a passion for living and communication that connects rather than harms.

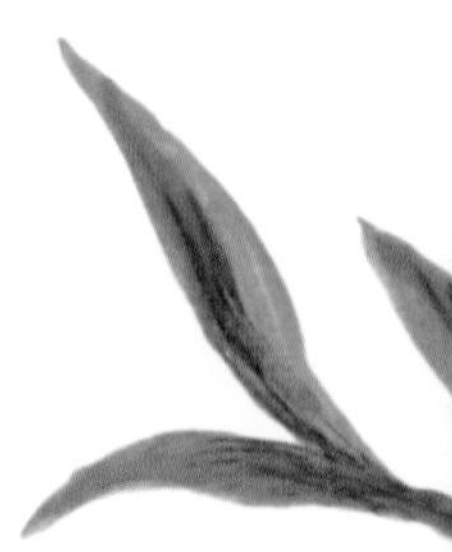

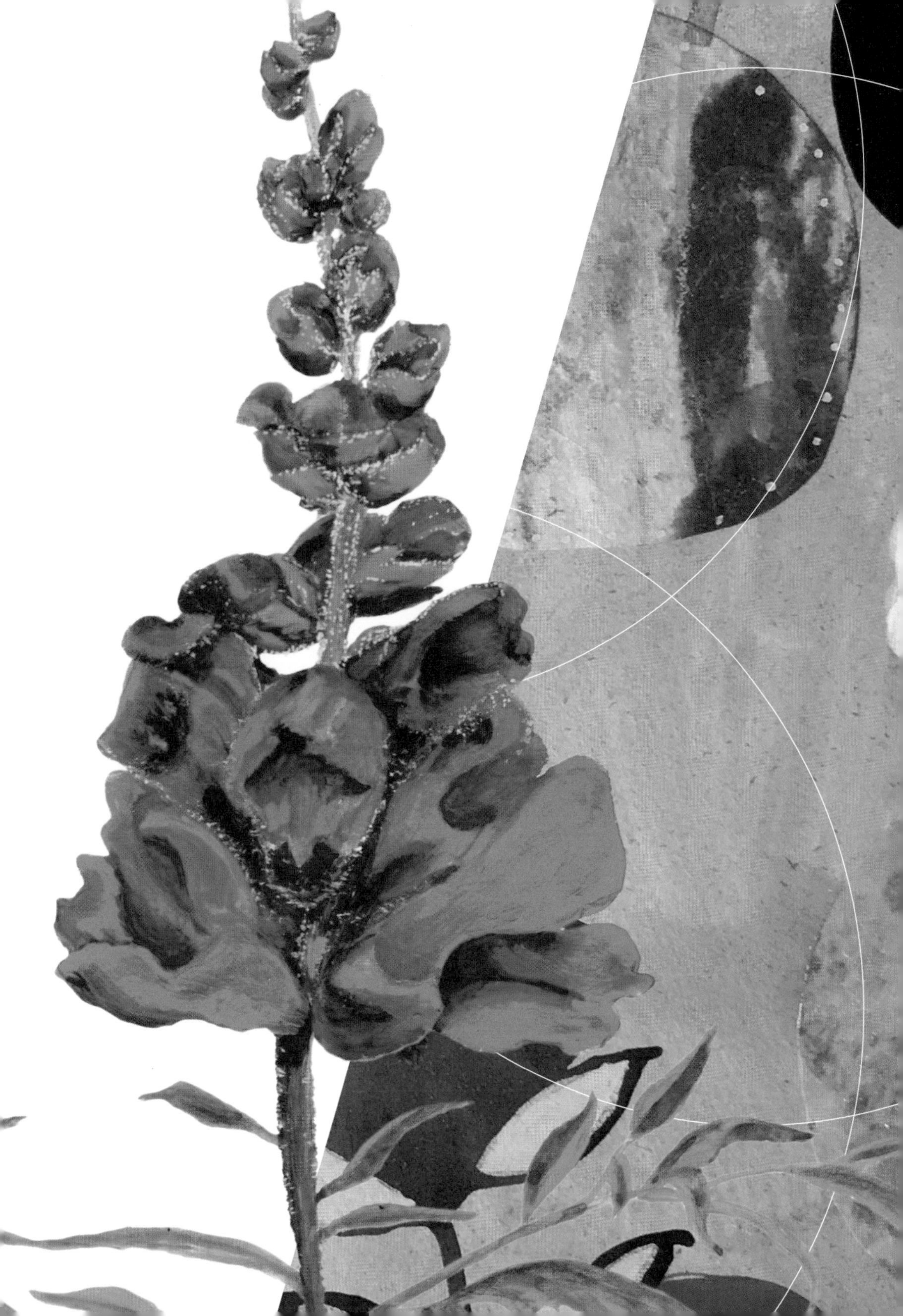

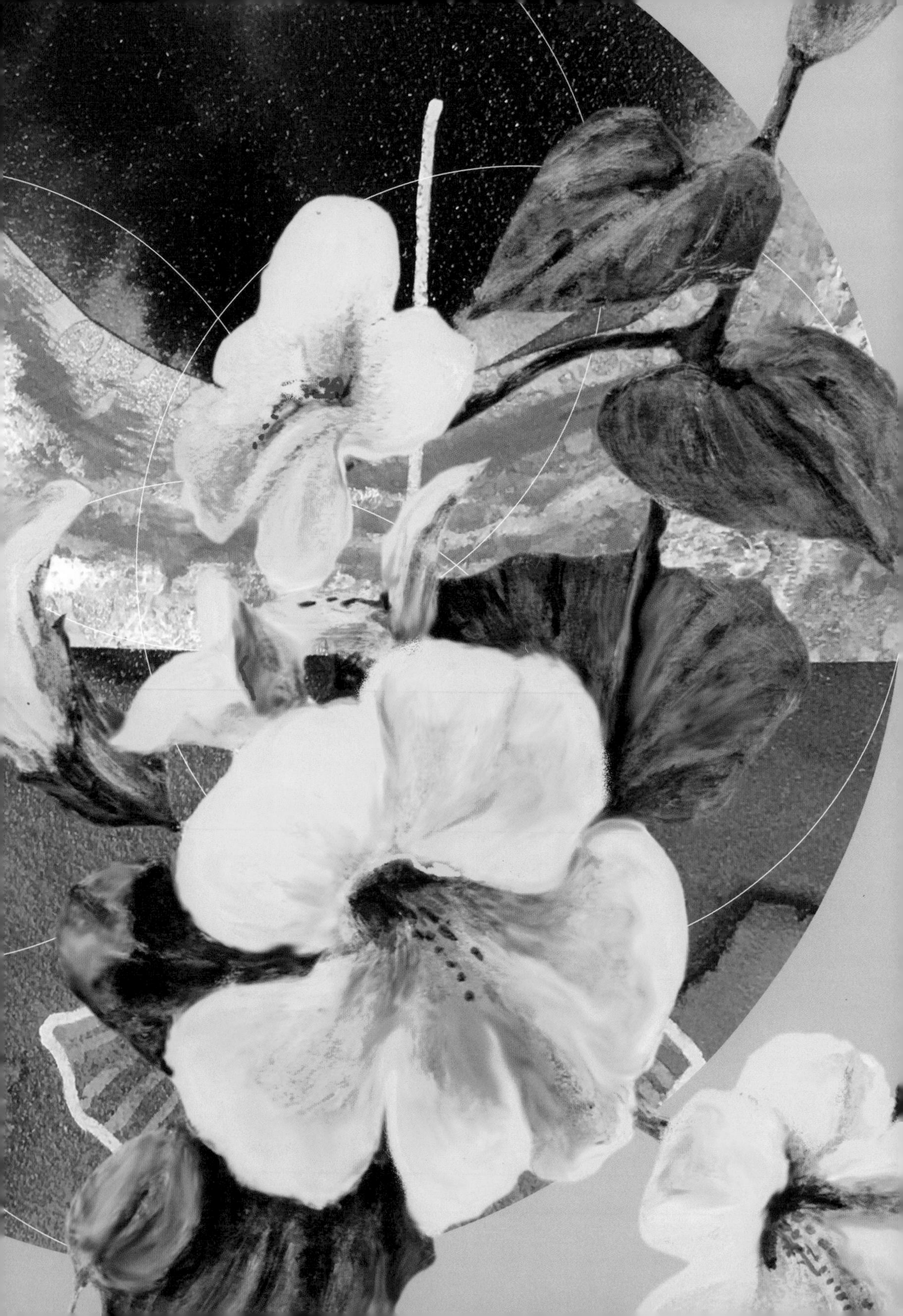

15 Interviews with Flower Essence Practitioners

"

The fact that I can plant a seed and it becomes a flower, share a bit of knowledge and it becomes another's, smile at someone and receive a smile in return, are to me continual spiritual exercises.

— Leo F. Buscaglia

Throughout the world, you can find flower essence practitioners who share a deep love and reverence for the flower realm. The following interviews share a glimpse of what it's like to work with flowers as a sweet and powerful medium for integration and wellness. Perhaps you will be moved to see such a practitioner for your own healing, as each approaches it as an art as they receive guidance from the flowers. Further, as you begin to work with the flowers, you will form your own personal relationship with the flower essences and will notice how they bestow their own form of healing and love inside you. This may inspire you to share your formulas with others as well.

Interview with Joseph Aldo

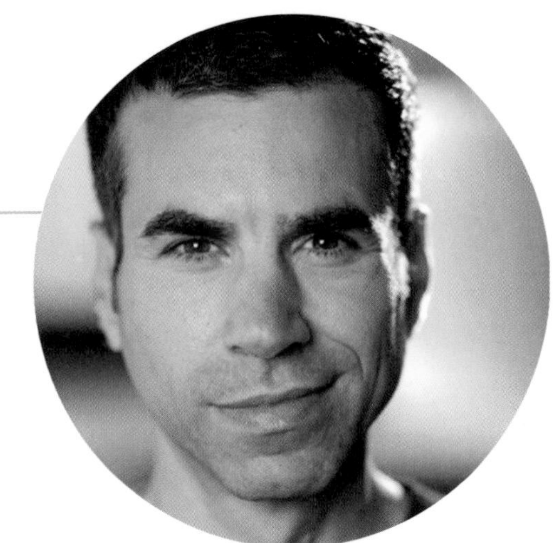

What drew you to become a flower essence practitioner? How long have you been working with the flowers?

My introduction to flower essences was when I working as an intuitive with Dr. Rudolph Ballentine (a holistic physician and author). He would prescribe flower essences to his clients, and when I saw the significant changes that the patients went through in such a short amount of time, my interest was piqued. I then began studying and giving flower essences to my clients with extraordinary results. I have been working with flower essences for more than twenty years.

Share some of your own experiences in working with and taking formulas.

I have been taking my own flower essence formulas for many years now. One of the most extraordinary experiences I had was when I woke up one morning at 3:00 a.m. with excruciating pain in my right side. It felt like my liver was swollen three times its size. So I communicated with my inner voice.

Within minutes I heard to take two flower essences: Crab Apple and Walnut. I slowly crawled (every move was so painful) to the cabinet that stored the essences and grabbed the two aforementioned remedies. When I got back into bed, I took one drop of each. Within five minutes the pain had subsided 50 percent. I took another drop of each essence after ten minutes and again, within five minutes, the pain had diminished another 40 percent. I took one more dose after ten minutes, fell asleep, and woke up hours later as if nothing had happened.

I asked my inner voice what that was all about, and it said, "Your father had a tumor in his hepatic flexure (right below the liver) and that tendency within your lineage to have such issues was just cleared." The Crab Apple relates to physical body issues, and Walnut helps cut the ties with the past. The Bach remedies helped me effectively and efficiently clear this lineage pattern and the problem has never returned (three years now).

I don't recommend that people take flower essences instead of going to the hospital when such a situation arises. However, because I am an intuitive and have many years of experience following my inner voice, as well as years of experience with energy medicine (flower essences and homeopathy), I had no doubt they could help in this situation. And sure enough, they did.

Regarding working with a client, I had a gentleman who came to me with his main issue being attention deficit disorder (ADD). He had been taking Western meds for his condition for more than fifteen years. He told me his symptoms, which included challenges staying focused, feeling ungrounded, always moving and fidgeting, impatience, and many fears, especially the fear of losing control (as if he would lose his mind). Intuitively, I could feel that there was some trauma related to this issue that needed to be addressed. The remedies I combined were Clematis for feeling ungrounded and his inability to stay focused; Impatiens for the impatience; Sweet Chestnut for the fear of losing control; Mimulus for known fears; Aspen for unknown fears; and Star of Bethlehem for the past trauma.

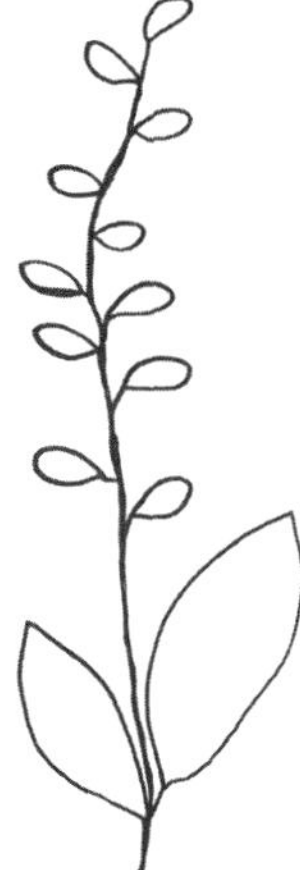

He returned a month later and informed me that he had stopped taking his meds the next day. "I no longer needed them," he said. "The flower essences made me feel so much calmer and brought more awareness of my relationship to my surroundings. I'm now able to be with people and feel much more grounded and present without spinning out of control. Also, the fear is much less."

I saw my client a year later at a music festival in town. He walked up to me and gave me a big hug. "I am doing great on the essences," he said, "and still medication free." Such words are music to my ears, words I hear often with the flower essences.

Do you have a favorite formula of your own, and why do you enjoy it?

My favorite formula is one that supports going through the Dark Night of the Soul. This is an experience that some people may go through when they are on a spiritual path, whereby the ego begins to dissolve and the personality identity is going through a massive change. From one day to the next, you can feel like the life you were living is no longer a viable option and that you must let go of your past and die to your former, limited self. I call it the evolutionary process of transforming from a caterpillar to a butterfly. The Dark Night of the Soul combo includes Aspen for unknown fears, Cherry Plum for the fear of losing control, Elm for feeling overwhelmed, Gorse for hopelessness and despair, Mustard for depression, Star of Bethlehem for shock, Sweet Chestnut for anguish and fear of going mad, and Walnut for letting go of the past.

This flower essence combination has helped me and many of my clients when going through transformative experiences that are filled with utter darkness and despair—as the ego tries to hold on to the familiar, albeit limiting, past. Anyone who is on a conscious path of evolution can expect to go through such a life-changing experience at some point in his or her life, and this remedy is gold.

What are some ways in which you connect to the flower realm?

I connect with the flowers by communing with Nature throughout the flowering months. I love going hiking, going to the Botanical Gardens, or simply walking through my neighborhood to see what new scents and sights Mother Nature has popping up.

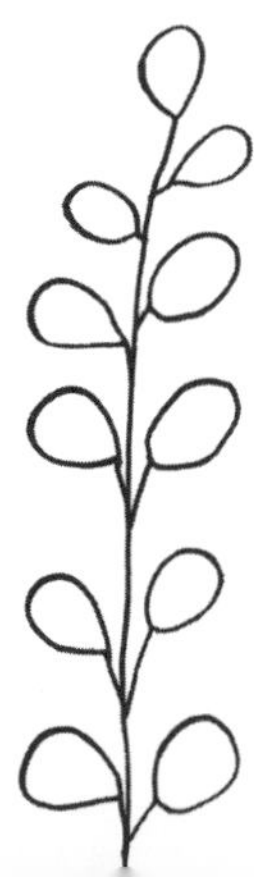

What can people expect once they begin integrating flower essences into their lives?

When taking flower essences, people can expect their lives to become much calmer and more peaceful as they support the release of old patterns, programs, and beliefs that underlie many of our emotional and psychological dis-eases. Issues of anger, grief, loneliness, insecurity, indecision, exhaustion, and many others can be resolved, oftentimes quickly, when bringing flower essences into one's life. Acute dosing in the moment can facilitate the integration of traumatic experiences from the past. This is one of the most extraordinary aspects of the flower essences I have experienced in my practice, one that leaves people dumbfounded as to how lifelong traumas can be addressed so quickly.

Share anything else that feels pertinent to you in regard to our flower friends.

Dr. Bach gifted us with one of the most simple, elegant, profound, and effective forms of medicine on the planet. Upon first glance, it would seem a bit incredulous that something so subtle as flower essences can have the capacity to effect such significant change. But I can assure you that after twenty-plus years of working with these wonderful healers, they can have a tremendous effect upon one's life. Direct experience is the true test for effectiveness, and I can attest to their effectiveness as I have seen miraculous transformations time and time again.

I believe that every household should have a kit of the 38 Bach remedies (see page 13), and that every parent should learn about these magical essences so that they can offer them to their children as well as take them for themselves. The family life will be so much more balanced and peaceful and trips to the doctor could be minimized greatly. I am deeply indebted to Dr. Bach for bringing forth one of the most beautiful healing gifts into this world. They have helped me, my family, my clients, and my pets in so many ways.

How can people find you? What sort of healing modalities do you offer besides recommending flower essence formulas?

People can find me at www.josephaldo.com. I am an intuitive holistic healer, spiritual mentor, and holder of a PhD in natural health. I work mostly with psycho-emotional issues through the use of energy medicine (flower essences and homeopathy) as well as various tools and techniques to integrate the shadow aspects within our subconscious. I am also a teacher of transformational courses, including Bach flower essence therapy, the evolution of consciousness, holistic healing seminars, and more.

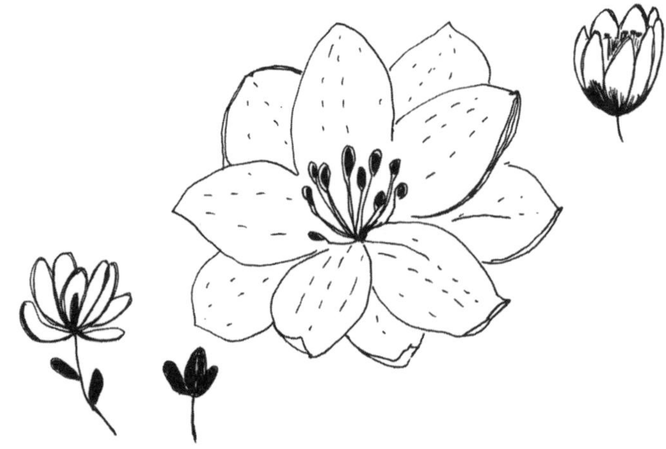

Interview with Kristina Crabtree

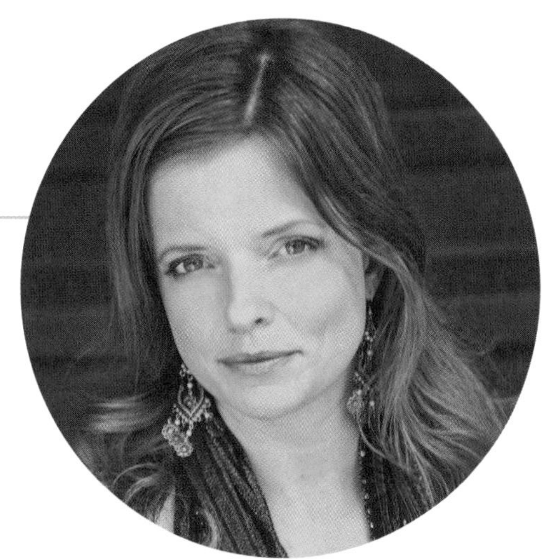

What drew you to becoming a flower essence practitioner? How long have you been working with the flowers?

I began working with flower essences more than a decade ago when I was studying herbalism in Asheville, North Carolina. I ended up feeling more drawn to connecting with and working with plants energetically. This was partly because my natural inclination is toward the subtle realms, and also because it is more sustainable at a time when overharvesting and industrialization have taken a toll on plant populations. It's a way to work with plant medicine and magick without requiring a ton of plant material, as with other supplements and essential oils, etc.

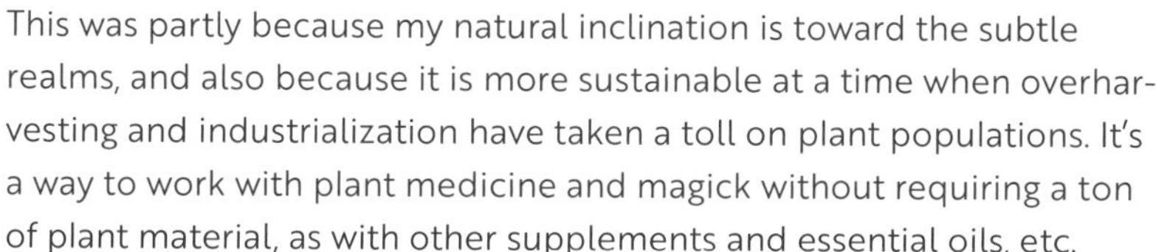

Share some of your own experiences in working with and taking formulas.

To me, flower essences feel like interdimensional friends. I have found the shifts to be so big when taking flower essences that I almost forget there was ever a problem. Like one time I was taking Mustard from the Bach essences and then just completely forgot that I had been depressed. My reality just shifted. It's like the essences recolor our world from the inside, like we put on a different pair of glasses. The change can seem so subtle.

Do you have a favorite formula of your own, and why do you enjoy it?

My biggest problem is I love them all and sometimes don't know where to start! I have really enjoyed Lotus and Star Tulip for opening the crown and connecting to cosmic energy, Corn for grounding, and Black Cohosh for healing. For clients, I create blends intuitively based on what shows up for them in a healing session. It is a good way to support the work they are doing in their lives with something they can take home and connect with daily.

What are some ways in which you connect to the flower realm?

My business name, Blomkraft, means "flower power" in Swedish. My favorite part of working with flower essences is making them, letting them infuse in pure water and sunlight! I loved traveling in India because they have fresh flowers as a part of daily life and ritual worship. They are always available, even in the most remote places! In my daily life, I keep fresh flowers around as much as possible; I think it is an important ritual to upgrade the energy of a space. Flowers speak to me in a holy language. Each one has such a special message for those who can tune in to their song, and the vibration they transmit is a true gift and reflection of our own higher nature!

What can people expect once they begin integrating flower essences into their lives?

Sometimes the shifts can be incredibly profound, so much so that you don't even notice! It's like the issue just dissolves. Sometimes you may feel everything, but it's like having a friend to hold your hand through the healing.

Share anything else that feels pertinent to you in regard to our flower friends.

Flower essences are transmitters of divine intelligence brought to you through form. They offer a way of communing with the subtle realms in a personalized manner. They are sacred teachers!

How can people find you? What sort of healing modalities do you offer besides recommending flower essence formulas?

I am based out of Asheville, North Carolina, and I can be found online at www.blomkraftstudio.com. I offer transformational healing sessions that include mantra and flower essences and am a licensed esthetician offering holistic beauty rituals and facials!

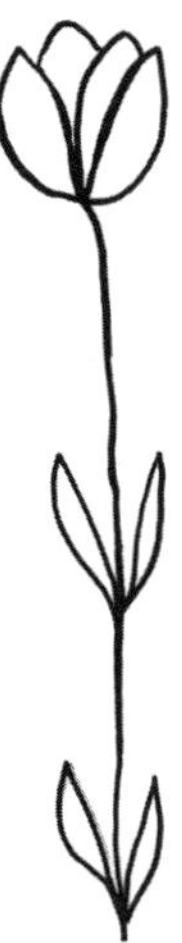

Interview with Daisy Marquis

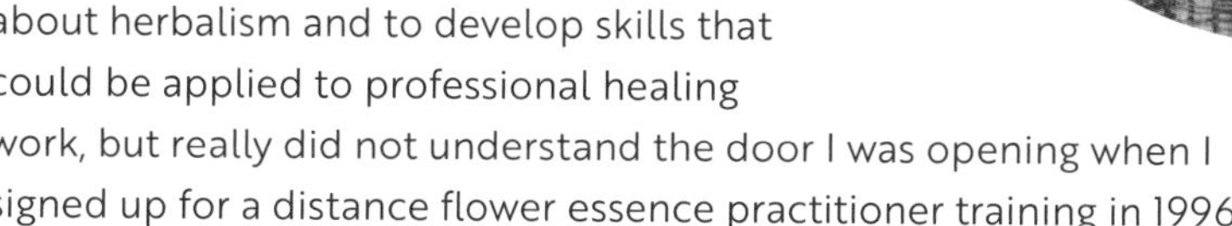

What drew you to becoming a flower essence practitioner? How long have you been working with the flowers?

When I first started learning about flower essences, they were a complete unknown to me. I was looking for ways to learn more about herbalism and to develop skills that could be applied to professional healing work, but really did not understand the door I was opening when I signed up for a distance flower essence practitioner training in 1996.

Share some of your own experiences in working with and taking formulas.

As part of that original distance training, I was given a flower essence formula—my first—and they began changing me immediately. I remember that formula included Crab Apple and Rescue Remedy, and three other Bach essences that I've forgotten now. It took about two weeks to notice a shift. It was subtle and gentle. The first observable change was decreased anxiety, decreased panic attacks. Over the years of working with flower essences therapeutically, I've had some dramatic awakenings and startling revelations, but most of the time the change that is brought about is very gentle and at the same time, marks a fundamental change in the way I relate to life.

Self-Heal was probably the most dramatic and sudden awakening experience that I've had. I took it for the first time right before bed and dreamed intensely vivid dreams about being on a trip with a man I'd been close friends with for years. In the dream we were camping on Mangrove roots with another woman. He began paying more and more attention to her, and less to me. The dream highlighted my internal decision-making process—to be quietly myself and observe the way they were connecting, or to change my behavior in a way that would grab his attention. I woke up in a state of extreme dismay, sobbing as if my heart had been broken. It had made undeniably clear all the ways

I had acted out of integrity in this relationship, in waking life, for years, being the person I thought my friend would value instead of my authentic self. I was devastated in seeing this part of myself so clearly, and at the same time, catapulted onto a path of healing and authenticity that is still alive in my consciousness today, twenty years later. This is how I came to understand that Self-Heal increases self-awareness and through doing so, helps us to be more responsible and to have a higher integrity in our actions. It helps us understand our own motivations.

Do you have a favorite formula of your own, and why do you enjoy it?

I usually work with flower essences singly, because I find it allows me to experience the individual nature of the plant in an intimate and clear way. I do value synergy! And I often recommend combinations to others, but find I lean toward one-on-one relationships in my inner work.

What are some ways in which you connect to the flower realm?

I connect with flowers by smelling them, taking photos of them, painting them, studying their historical and modern applications as herbal medicines, making medicines with them, reading poetry about them, holding them while meditating so that I can feel their subtle effects in my body, and asking them questions. I also love to just gaze in wonder at flowers and tell them how beautiful and amazing they are! The most important thing in cultivating a relationship with flowers, though, is to become very quiet and still inside yourself. The voice of the flowers is so quiet. If your own mind is busy, loud, or overstimulated, you'll have a much more difficult time tuning in to them.

What can people expect once they begin integrating flower essences into their lives?

Working with flower essences awakens wonder and respect for the incredible and immeasurable intelligence present in the natural world, first and foremost. Having the direct experience of the transformative power and the all-encompassing compassion of the flowers changes a person forever. Life's magick becomes apparent. And then you're never again able to ignore the living, conscious presence that inhabits every aspect of nature. You become humble and grateful.

How can people find you? What sort of healing modalities do you offer besides prescribing formulas?

I am currently only working through distance-based, one-on-one teaching and can be found mostly through the Facebook page for the Black Mountain School of Natural Healing, and through direct referral.

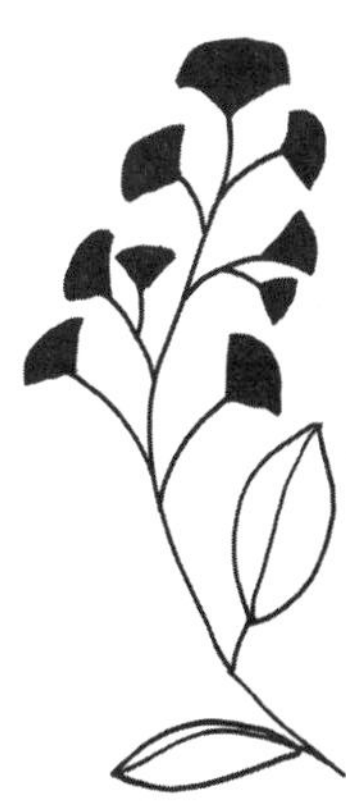

Interview with Lupo Lauren Passero

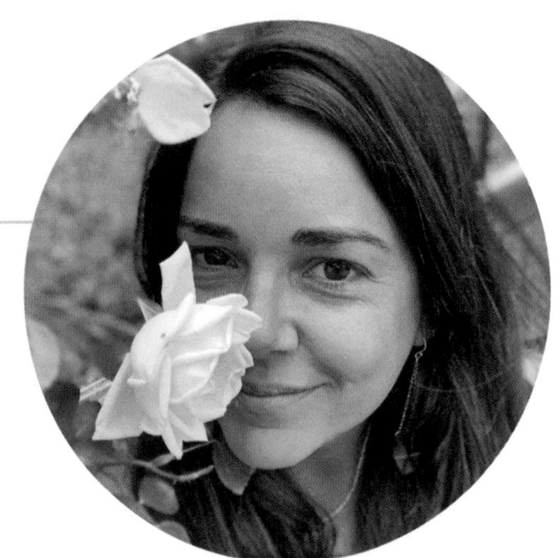

What drew you to becoming a flower essence practitioner? How long have you been working with the flowers?

My passion for flower essences stemmed from my initial studying of herbal medicine, in which I formally began training when I was twenty-one years old. I was completely enamored with all of the different aspects of healing that plants had to offer. As a part of one of my early herbal trainings, we learned about flower essences. Having always considered myself to be incredibly sensitive and highly emotional, I was totally blown away when I found out that there were remedies that could help support these emotions and sensitivities. To me this felt like the greatest gift. I have always had an innate belief that physical illness oftentimes has an emotional component attached to it, so when I learned that the flower essences help heal emotional traumas and dramas, these remedies became the perfect pairing along with healing herbs.

A few years later, when I went on to become a clinical herbalist and I began to see my first clients, not only did I find myself recommending different types of herbal formulations, but I also always recommended a flower essence blend. Each client that I saw or person I worked with (including myself) seemed to have an emotional issue or response that was impeding upon their physical health. This seemed particularly true with folks who were dealing with long-term or chronic illnesses. The magical part was that when clients would walk into the room to see me and they would begin to share their story, oftentimes the flowers would just pop into my head.

Often prior to the consultation I would think about a particular flower, or after arriving the person would remind me of a flower, and sure enough, after some research, I would find that those very remedies were perfectly indicated for them. I learned early on how to trust my own intuition and also to trust messages the plants send to us, when we are open to it. For the last twenty-plus years, I have been working with flower essences, as a consultant, teacher, and representative of some of the finest flower essences in the world. I recommend them to all of my clients, my students, and my apothecary customers. And I cannot imagine having successfully raised two amazing children without them.

Share some of your own experiences in working with and taking formulas.

The greatest thing that I can share was the very first time I had what I like to refer to as an "aha" moment with the essences. I had been working with them for several years, finding success with both myself and with clients. When I first began to work with Pine, that is when I felt such a tremendous shift within myself that was so tangible that I was never the same again. Taking that essence for just a few days had an immediate effect and released me from a lifelong history of dealing with an all-too-familiar negative emotion, guilt. I had just had my second child and was in my early twenties. After her birth I suffered from postpartum depression, and with that came a lot of guilt and shame. Feelings that I have had since I was a child myself and I never really dealt with. I decided that I didn't want to pass these qualities on to my daughter, and it was time for me to let go of the particular feelings that were holding me back and making me physically ill.

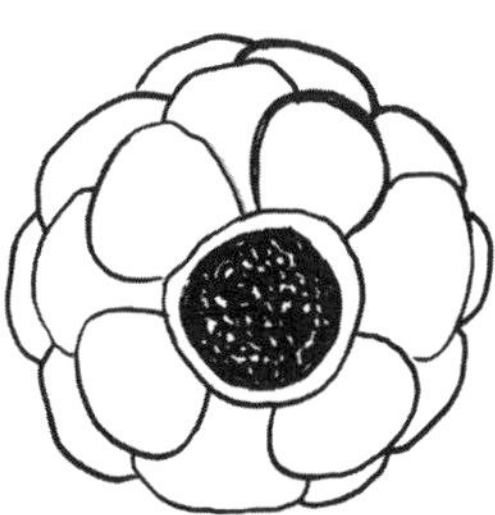

I started taking Pine flower essence, and within three days felt an immediate shift. All of the guilt that I had learned to carry and take on as a child, and had carried with me into my adult life, suddenly vanished. I no longer felt like I was a bad person, and I was able to let go of the religious ideals that I had been raised with that had been so detrimental to my health and well-being. I was free of these feelings for the first time in my life, and they did not return after that. It was by far one of the most profound experiences I've ever had with any type of plant remedy, and I will be forever changed and grateful.

Do you have a favorite formula of your own, and why do you enjoy it?

I don't have a particular favorite formula that I work with, as I believe it is important to make personalized remedies for the individual and have found that no two personalities or formulas are ever the same. I have, however, found certain remedies that pair really well together that I tend to use often in similarly themed formulas. Elm, Oak, and Pink Yarrow are the first to come to mind. The Oak personality, or the individual who would benefit from Oak essences, tends to take on too much, which often leads to feelings of overwhelm. Elm essence is perfectly indicated for easing feelings of overwhelm. I find that the two of these essences are often needed at the same time. The individual who takes on too much or becomes too easily overwhelmed often has a sensitive personality and an empathic heart that is often the cause. Pink Yarrow helps support the emotional self as well as the heart and helps us set better boundaries for ourselves and learn not to take on other people's energies or pain.

I also tend to pair Walnut and Corn essence together for folks who need to feel grounded and embodied. Walnut, like Pink Yarrow, is a protective essence that allows us to feel sure of ourselves throughout transition. Corn offers a close connection to the earth and trust in oneself. This combination is often indicated for folks who cannot seem to stay grounded. Shooting Star is another essence that I may add to a grounding formula, particularly for those who feel like they don't belong here or cannot connect to their environment.

For addiction issues, I tend to pair Agrimony, Willow, and Nicotiana, whether it be for drugs, alcohol, food, tobacco, or any other vice that one may have that is not serving one. Agrimony is perfectly indicated for folks who hide behind their addictions, preventing emotional honesty and allowing the substances to hide their true feelings. Willow is a beautiful essence for letting go of pain and resentments, which often lead to our addictions in the first place. And Nicotiana is indicated for those searching for inner peace and emotional well-being. I also tend to put Rock Water in most formulas, as many of us need to be reminded to relinquish control and surrender to the process, as well as Self-Heal, which is a gentle reminder for self-care and a nice way for folks to remember to take their essences!

What are some ways in which you connect to the flower realm?

I connect with the flower realm via my deep and personal relationship with flowers, which stems from considering all plant beings both family and friends and treating them as such. Talking to them, sitting with them, photographing and drawing them, collecting them, and making remedies with them are just a few ways of connecting with them. I constantly find myself complimenting their beauty aloud, and more than anything giving thanks and gratitude prayers for their giving spirits and for their precious medicine. I believe that relationships with plants and flowers are no different than those with humans or animals. It just takes time to cultivate and develop them. Once that relationship is established, you have made a lifelong friend or plant ally that can be called upon at any time. I find that paying attention to the language of the flower and allowing it to show us what its medicine is, is the surest way to build the right relationships with the flower and plant realm.

What can people expect once they begin integrating flower essences into their lives?

Again, no two experiences are ever quite the same. Sometimes the essence works in subtle ways that you may not notice until weeks or months later. Other times it has an immediate effect with only a few dosages. Regardless of the immediate experience, the essences work to usher out the negative emotions or experiences that may be standing in the way of our healing. They flood the body with positive attributes and energies meant to gently wash away negative energies or influences that may need to be released. Sometimes in this release process, folks may experience an emotional response, either positive or negative, but usually not more than the person can handle. It is important to pay attention to your thoughts, feelings, and emotions when taking the essences—particularly if you are working on a deep-seated or long-standing trauma. It is important to be gentle with oneself and allow proper time for self-care and reflection.

Share anything else that feels pertinent to you in regard to our flower friends.

I have found the essences to be such a profound part of my own life as an herbalist, a flower essences practitioner, and a mother. And hundreds, if not thousands, of times I have witnessed the healing ability of these remedies helping relieve folks of suffering and uncovering pertinent parts of their healing process that no other modalities could touch. These remedies are gentle yet powerful, and no others can compare. They offer us true soul healing and can wash away and transform pain, fear, grief, and more while supporting us on our healing path. They are gentle yet effective, often being the key or missing piece to unresolved or stubborn issues in the body. This method of healing is well worth learning more about and can easily be paired with other healing practices. It does take time to get to know and fully understand the essences, and just like any relationship, the longer you are in it, the more profound it becomes. I believe it is well worth the time and energy to spend with the remedies and getting to know the healing power of the flowers.

How can people find you? What sort of healing modalities do you offer besides recommending formulas?

Folks can find me at Twin Star Herbal Education and Community Apothecary located in downtown New Milford, Connecticut, just an hour outside of New York City. We have a full herbal apothecary with hundreds of flower essences and offer custom formulas and consultations in person, by phone, and online. Our apothecary is staffed with skilled herbalists and flower essence practitioners who can custom-blend teas, herbal tinctures, essences, and more. Through our certification school, we offer trainings, certifications, and retreats on flower essence therapy as well as herbalism, plant spirit healing, and more. We do not offer many online trainings, as we believe that this lineage of healing is meant to be shared in person; however, we do have one training on flower essence therapy for folks who do not have access to a local school or teacher. Please visit on Instagram at @twinstartribe or online at www.twinstartribe.com.

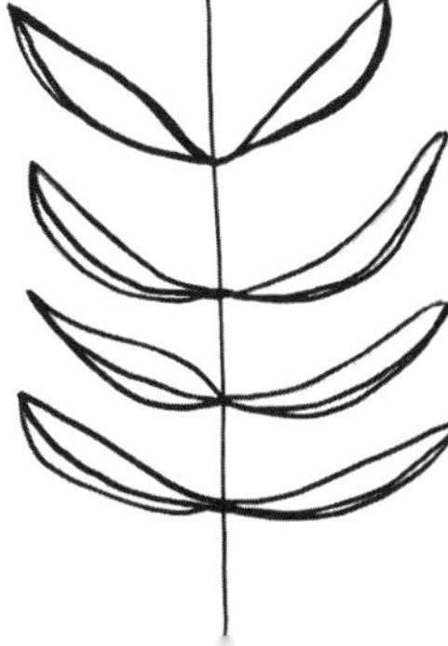

Interview with Lena Ruark-Eastes

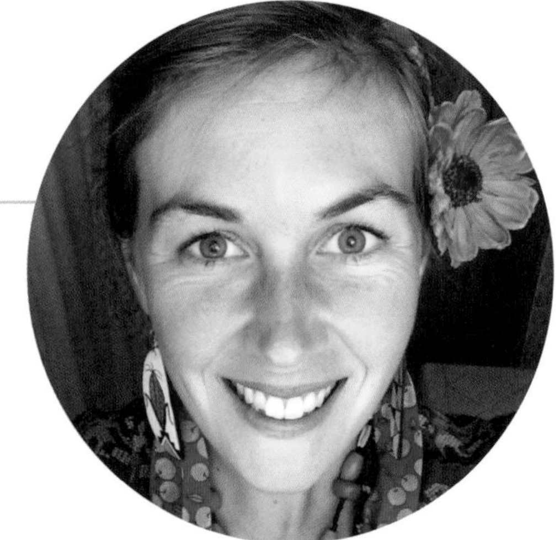

What drew you to becoming a flower essence practitioner? How long have you been working with the flowers?

As I child, before I even knew about flower essences, I would visit the flowers and sip the dew off their petals. It brought me ecstatic joy; it's instinctual. Fifteen years ago, I learned how to make my own flower essences, and that is where my practice really began. I love to teach young women how to make flower essences, and more importantly how to be in relation with flowers. Now I find myself surrounded by flowers, as I am a flower farmer and designer. I make altars with flowers, design wedding flowers, grow flowers, make essences, and have a healing practice with flower essences.

Share some of your own experiences in working with and taking formulas.

Pink Lady Slipper abounds near my home in the Appalachian Mountains, and I have an affinity for her medicine of aligning one with their highest purpose in this life and awakening one's path of embodied service. Pink Lady Slipper is one of my ally flowers and essences that I've worked with regularly for more than a decade. We're on a deep journey of living a spirit-led life right here and now in my temple of a body.

As a flower essence practitioner, I work in an intuitive way and bring my gift of deep listening and presence to both my client and the flowers. We always make both a spray and an oral application and also develop an accompanying prayer and intention to be taken with the essences.

Do you have a favorite formula of your own, and why do you enjoy it?

Yes, I'm all about my Find Your YES! Formula: Hibiscus, Sunflower, Cosmos, Pink Lady Slipper, Rose, and Lily. Through healthy sexual expression, radiating one's light, having healthy boundaries, knowing and using our No, and aligning with the Divine, you can Find Your YES!

What are some ways in which you connect to the flower realm?

Tending to the life cycle of the flower, from the corms, seeds, bulbs, and transplants, all the way to the flowering, to death and rebirth. As a flower farmer, I see flowers in all their seasons, and this connects me to them as cycling beings. It's a miracle every time a flower opens her face to the sun. I love to connect from my flower essence apothecary into my water, and into my Spirit, and I love to be with the living flowers in my garden and the forest. Here in Appalachia, we're blessed with an abundance of wildflowers, and I enjoy meditating and talking with these wise beings.

What can people expect once they begin integrating flower essences into their lives?

A softening, a grace, potent healing by addressing one's truth layer by layer. Feeling uplifted and beautiful; an increase in self-love and care. A blossoming in one's heart.

Share anything else that feels pertinent to you in regard to our flower friends.

It's about relationships. Yes, start with books, start with sets of essences and with practitioners, and also remember they are speaking to you too. You can always go directly to a flower and introduce yourself and listen. Listen directly to the wisdom of the flower and your personal connection. It's you and a flower as individuals who have gifts for one another. How can you be a gift to the flowers?

How can people find you? What sort of healing modalities do you offer besides recommending flower essence formulas?

I offer Nature Based Rites of Passage for Young Women and Rites of Passage Guide trainings, along with ceremonial flowers, flowers designed for your ceremony, customized essences of your wedding flowers, flower essence sessions, and more. You can find me online at www.earthpatheducation.com.

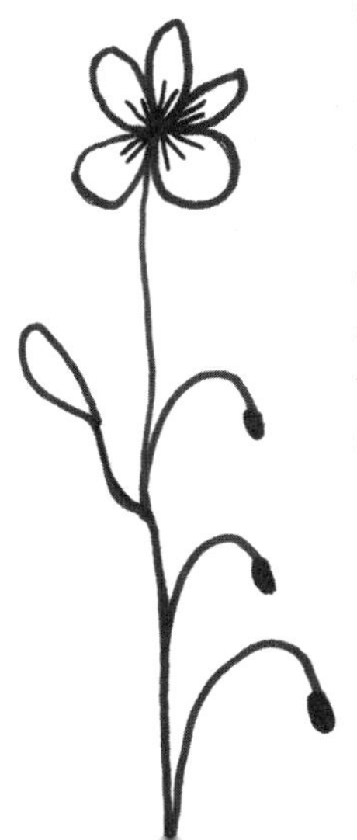

Interview with Asia Suler

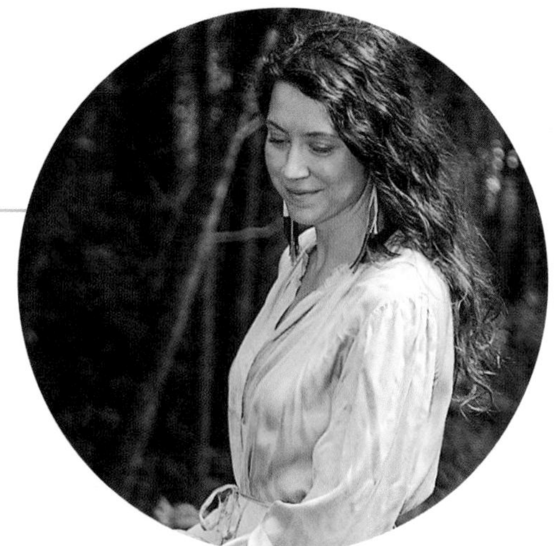

What drew you to becoming a flower essence practitioner? How long have you been working with the flowers?

Way back before I even knew what herbalism was, I stumbled across a book about the Bach flower remedies. I had no idea what the book was about, but I was curious about plants, so I brought it home to peruse. I still remember the night I began reading. It stands out vividly in my mind as a moment that changed my life. Reading it was like stumbling across a whole way of seeing the world that gave words to something I had always felt but never fully realized. By the end of the introduction, I was crying. I wasn't sad or overwhelmed; I wasn't even awed. I was crying because what I read—about the vibrational nature of reality, a flower's ability to help us heal, and the inner blocks we erect that stunt our incredible blossoming—struck me so deeply as reality, I couldn't help but weep. I call these tears "truth cries" now, and I recognize moments when they come as one of my most potent guides. I started working with flower essences soon after that. To date I've been working with their medicine for a decade, and I still have truth cries arise when I stumble upon just the right essence at the right time.

Share some of your own experiences in working with and taking formulas.

I see formula-making as a deeply intuitive practice. To me, we are a part of the formula as a whole, so when I'm creating a blend, I hold not just the combination of flowers in my mind, but also myself (or the client) as an actual element in the formula itself. A given combination might make sense for one client but, like a tuning fork that is slightly off-key, when I substitute one person for another, the whole thing falls slightly flat. The same goes for trying out different essences. I keep feeling into the various combinations, as if creating a perfume with the perfect blend of notes, almost undetectable before it all comes together, until the formula transforms from a combination of singles into an entire whole. Formulas are alchemical by nature. The elements of the formula come together in order to transform the whole. In esoteric alchemy, the goal is not to turn base metal into gold, but to help our own spirit transform into the fullest expression of ourselves. Flower essence formulas initiate an alchemy of the spirit, a kind of transformation that is akin to the eternal blossoming of gold.

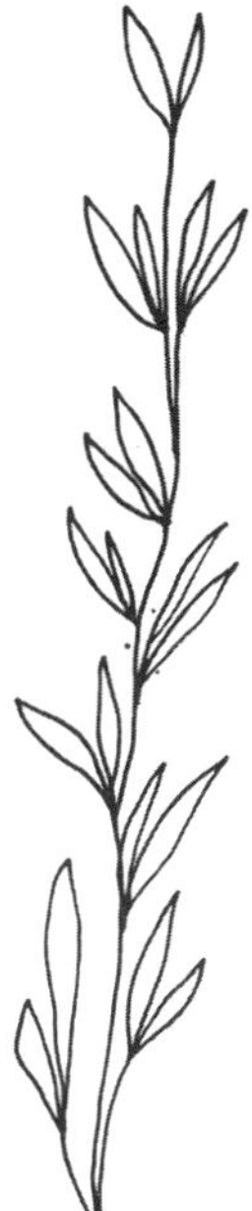

Do you have a favorite formula of your own, and why do you enjoy it?

I tend to make formulas for very specific periods of time in my life, and then let them go. I always tell my clients to take a formula, or a single essence, until they forget to take it one day—that is when they know they are done with that arc of healing. I've made formulas for a particular travel adventure, for the beginning of new relationships, for the end of relationships, for times of great change in my business, and for anxiety, excitement, or loss. I give them a name that is emblematic of how I want to feel at that moment in my life, so just seeing them on my counter empowers me. Each one is special, and I tend to not repeat them once they are done. That said, if I had to choose, I might say my favorite formula to date is a combination of a flower and a stone—Self-Heal and mica—two medicines that are spectacularly good at helping us see ourselves clearly and with uncompromising compassion. I often take this formula with me to gift to the waters of any landscape I'm visiting, and it always feels so deeply good to give back to the earth.

What are some ways in which you connect to the flower realm?

Growing flowers is my favorite way to really get to know a given bloom. If I can't grow a flower, I try to visit the blossom every day over its period of flowering. A single flower doesn't tend to be in bloom for a very long time (though an entire plant can bloom all season, and some flowers are hardier than others). Just like a lifelong friend, you learn so much from seeing a flower move through its transition from bud, to peak, to waning. If you are truly lucky, then you might even be able to keep watching as it moves into seed and fruit. Once you see a flower move through its whole life-death transition, you will never forget it, or its medicine.

What can people expect once they begin integrating flower essences into their lives?

One of the biggest things I've noticed with beginning to take flower essences is the increased ability to be attuned to the subtle. Flower essences, like most vibrational medicine, are both subtle and powerful; their power lies in their subtlety. Often, the most healing experiences with flower essences will seem to take place almost behind the scenes. Like any natural healing, one day you'll look back and wonder at where you used to be, because the transformation into who you are now will have been so graceful. That said, beginning to take a flower essence has the incredible ability to open us up to noticing subtleties. The subtle realms are where all the best magick happens—the differences in the colors of the forest, the scent of two different roses, the knowledge of what is intuition versus anxiety, or that tingly wave of wonder that precedes a moment of deep insight. Being attuned to subtlety also helps us notice when we first begin to feel "off," and to address it as it comes up. Conversely, knowing how to sense and interact with subtleties can also open up so many layers of beauty, pleasure, magick, and perception. The subtle realm is the same as the spiritual realm, or the realm of consciousness. Just by beginning to work with flower essences, all these worlds start to open up for people.

Share anything else that feels pertinent to you in regard to our flower friends.

I think flower essence books, or written descriptions, are lovely. But I always tell people to trust what they hear from a given flower. Every description of a flower essence is just something that a flower once whispered in a particular person's ear. It is not the only account of that flower's healing capabilities—far from it. We are in a time in which it is increasingly necessary that we all enact our ability to speak to the more-than-human world and bring its multileveled wisdom into our libraries of shared knowledge. I always encourage my students to think about the attunement process with a flower essence as an interview. Just like in any interview, you will never hear every single detail about a person. What that person tells you will depend on who you are, where you are coming from, and what questions you ask. So please know that if you receive something from a flower essence that is different than what has been written about before, you aren't wrong, you are actually helping us all by bringing more diverse knowledge to the whole. Your experience with flower essences is a part of nurturing the well of our collective knowledge and is a gift that you can give to the world.

How can people find you? What sort of healing modalities do you offer besides recommending flower essence formulas?

To learn more about my work with herbalism, earth connection, intuition, flower essences, stone medicine, vaginal healing, and animism, find me over on my website, www.onewillowapothecaries.com. As a gathering place for healing and education, the site includes videos, writings, online classes, apothecary products, and information about my in-person retreats. You can also find me over at YouTube, on Facebook, and on Instagram @onewillow_apothecaries.

Interview with Brooke Sullivan

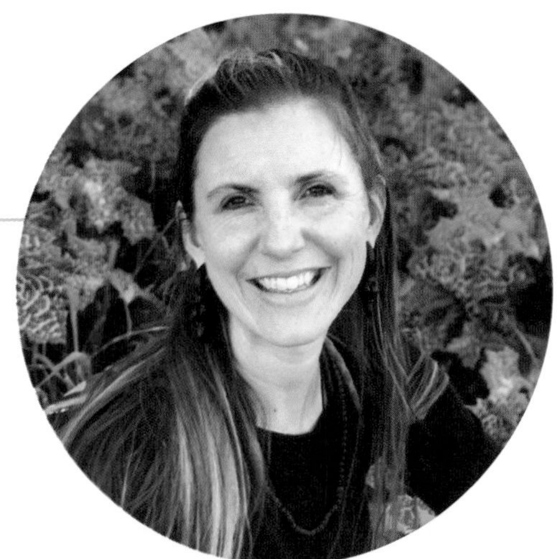

What drew you to becoming a flower essence practitioner? How long have you been working with the flowers?

When I was pregnant almost two decades ago, I was also in midwifery school studying homeopathy. My passion was the psychology of the remedies, which I happened to have a knack for. I started to support my family and community with what I was learning. Around this time, a dear friend of mine gave me the complete Bach Flower Essence set and the *Flower Essence Repertory* "Bible" and said, "Hey, you should check this out; I think you would like it." She did not have the time or interest, and she was hoping I would help support her family with the gems of what I learned. This was one of the biggest unknown-at-the-time blessings I have ever received.

Share some of your own experiences in working with and taking formulas.

As a Simpler, one who likes to get to know a plant deeply and work one at a time in building relationships to the plants, I prefer to take essences one at a time. However, when people come to me for flower essence therapy, I often do simple blends—usually a trinity—so they can get to know the flowers better, as well as have supporting essence to better direct the healing or to support them in moving through the healing. Too many essences in a formula, in my opinion, can be too complex. It also doesn't always empower the client to connect with each flower. The flowers have particular medicine that is evolving as we evolve, and they carry an intelligence that is close to spirit. Their work can be mysterious. Often just one flower essence with an intention, as long as it is the right essence at that time, has all a person needs for a huge transformational healing.

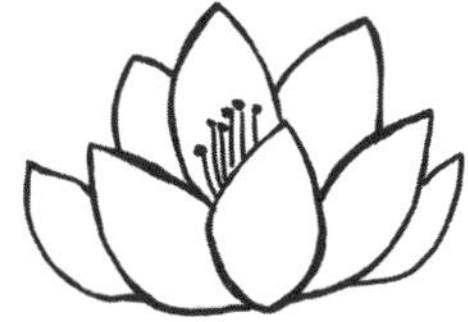

Do you have a favorite formula of your own, and why do you enjoy it?

With all that said above, I have two that I have seen working for a particular pattern of clients for almost twenty years.

My favorite formula is a trinity blend for empaths. It works amazingly. It is Pink Yarrow, Corn for grounding, and Walnut. The formula works so well because often people don't realize they are empaths, and taking it helps them not "bleed out their life blood" into others, nor absorb toxic emotions and vibes like a psychic sponge. The Corn helps ground and connect to Mother Earth, which helps mentally as well as physically (in times of stress and sympathetic overdrive). The Walnut acts as a shield sanctuary for the person to be not only solidly in their own field of energy but also to disconnect the psychic cords and even ideas of others that can be toxic. White Yarrow is very similar to Walnut in this action, but I love Walnut in this formula, as it also brings one into their next stage of evolution, which is great for empaths who have perhaps been dealing with this pathology for years.

My other favorite formula (and first, and therefore oldest formula) is for teachers and people who have to speak in public, due to their profession. Larch for the confidence to Speak and to Do YOU, Trumpet Vine for the eloquence in doing so, White Yarrow to keep your aura "tight" (meaning not being influenced so much by others' thoughts and impressions), and Cosmo for pulling inspiration down from Universal Consciousness and weaving this inspiration to create your own thoughts/ideas.

What are some ways in which you connect to the flower realm?

Being in my heart space and creative mode is often what connects me most to the flower realm. I am also a meditator and plant lover, so whenever I see a plant or I am in nature, I notice them. I believe my knowledge of who they are or curiosity of who they are begins a green language between us. When I want or need to do deep relationship work (plant study) with a plant, I first sit or stand, let my thoughts wash away, and presence myself with this being. I may say hello, make an offering of a song, and talk to them. I often spill over my gratitude every time I see an old friend or new potential that calls me, which is also why I think they "call out to me" often.

Connecting to the green world is really about listening and observing. Paracelsus taught us that. Often my observation involves drawing the plants and journaling what thoughts arise as I do so. I also listen to my dreams, as the plants often find me in that space, and I learn from them a lot there!

What can people expect once they begin integrating flower essences into their lives?

I feel that weaving the flower essences into one's life is an incredible gift of what is possible outside of our mundane, material world. On the inside, feelings such as peace, confidence, or forgiveness we have never before felt, arise. This is quite an awakening, and quite healing. On the outside, we become more present. We start to feel awe and a deeper connection with the natural world. This connection is truly a panacea in our modern time of such disconnect, as it makes us really see nature's beauty, creates a desire to take care of nature more, and overall makes us feel good—that we belong.

Share anything else that feels pertinent to you in regard to our flower friends.

What I have realized is, to really get to know a plant, tend to it. Grow it in your garden, have houseplants, or visit plants in the wild. You can get deep, sustaining healing from taking them out of the bottle, but to truly connect to the plants and understand their medicine, magick, and mystery, be with them.

How can people find you? What sort of healing modalities do you offer besides prescribing formulas?

I currently live in Northern California and run a school called The Wild Temple, which offers professional trainings in yoga therapy, yoga teacher training, herbalism, and flower essence wisdom. I am currently writing a book on spiritual herbalism, so stay in touch with me! You can find me on Instagram under @thewildtemple or on Facebook as Brooke Sullivan. My school has two Facebook pages, The Wild Temple School of Herbal Wisdom and also a flower essence group, The Wild Temple Flower Essences. I lead annual retreats to England (and the Bach Centre, along with all things magical and Avalon), Mount Shasta, Ireland, and India, and all of my adventures are a weave of plants and yoga.

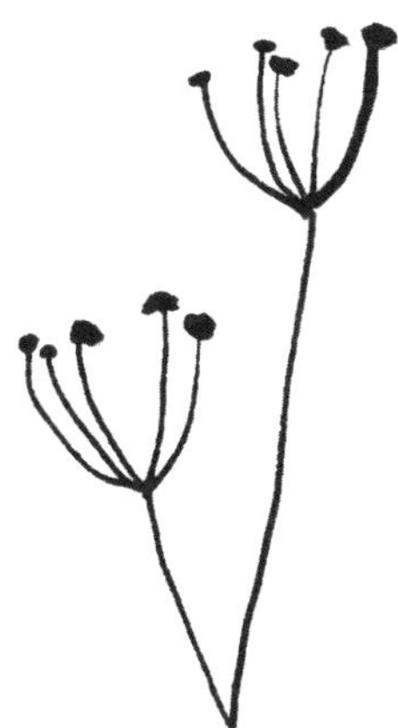

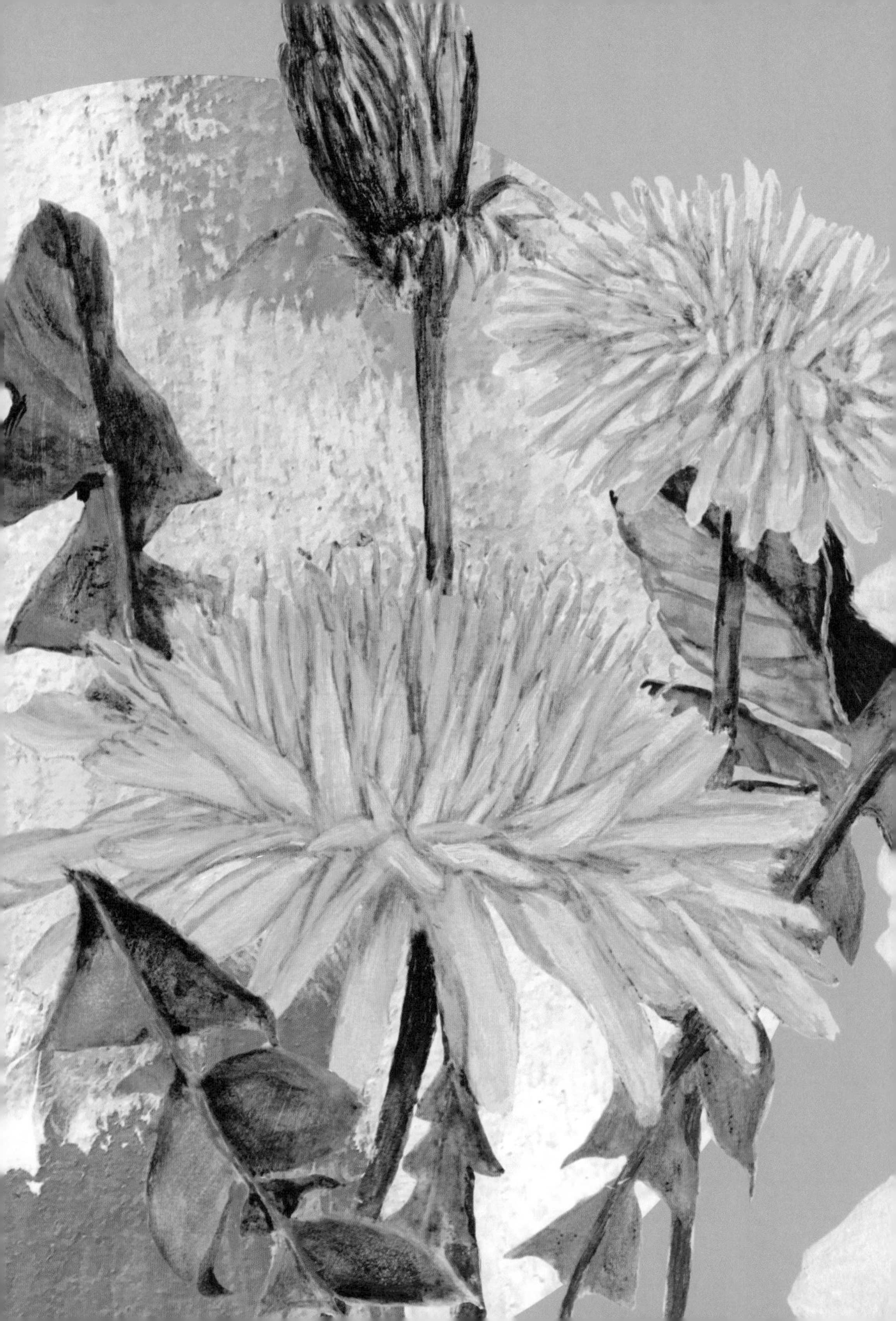

Resources

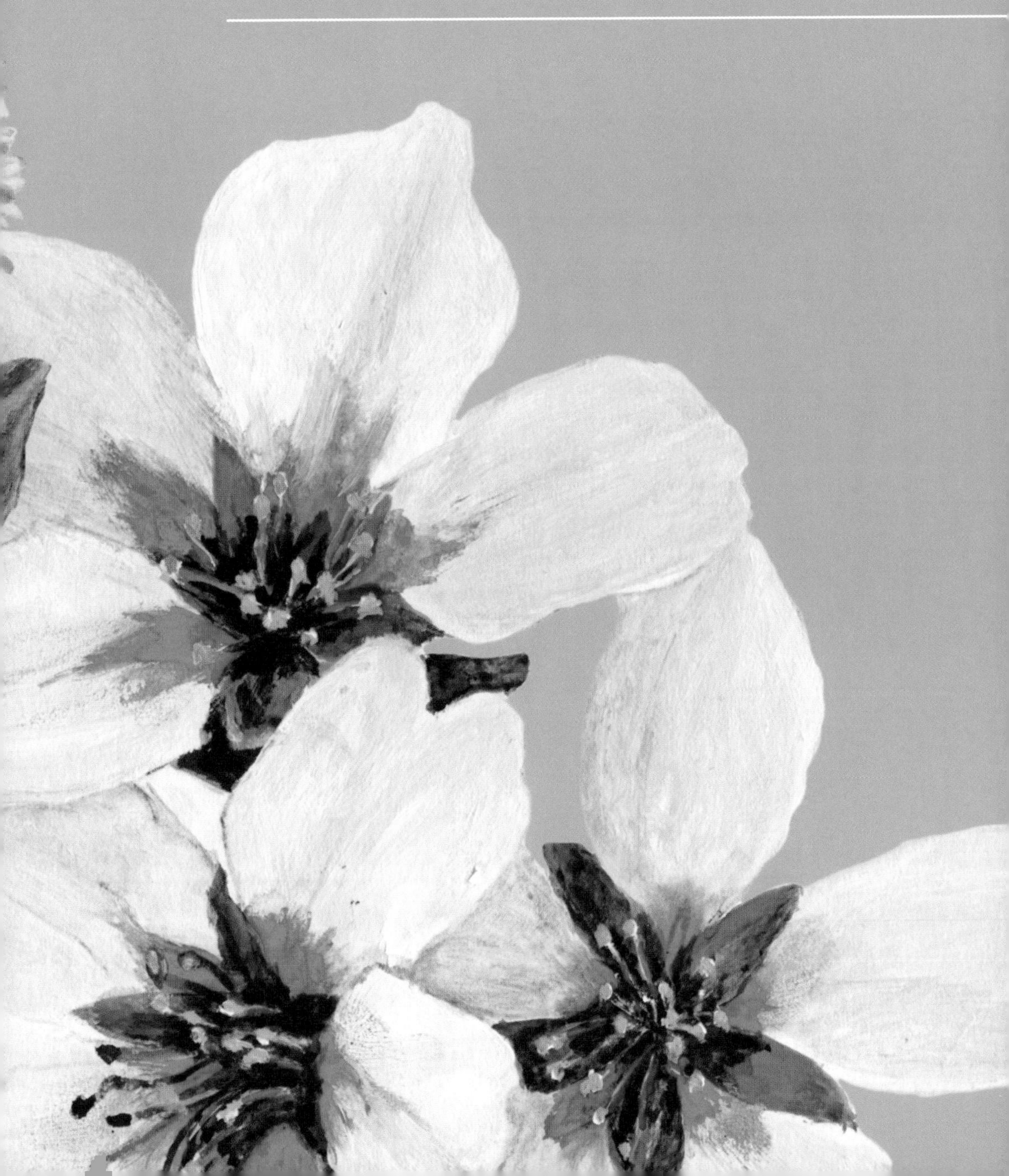

How to Become a Certified Flower Essence Practitioner

There are a variety of ways you can study, receive, and work with the flowers to become a flower essence practitioner yourself. You can attend workshops in person or online. The Bach Centre created a four-level course to become a Bach Foundation Registered Practitioner. You can learn in person at Dr. Bach's home in Oxfordshire, England; at any Bach Centre–approved location; or by signing up for the distance-learning program, which is done through email. It is possible, with intent, to complete all four levels of training within twelve months. Learn more at www.bachcentre.com.

The Flower Essence Society (FES) also offers trainings to become a practitioner, through their FES Practitioner Certification Program. The prerequisite is completion of the FES Professional Course, which is held in Nevada City, California. This is a special opportunity for theoretical and experiential learning onsite at FES. The FES Practitioner Certification Program is a poststudy option that provides opportunities for case studies with individuals or animals and flower remedies. Learn more at www.flowersociety.org.

Alaskan Essences offers a comprehensive Practitioner Training Program in the United States, Japan, and Brazil. Each program requires in-person training as well as case study findings. The training provides theory, practice, and experience. Each training is held in a stunningly beautiful setting of rich plant habitats for seven days. Alaskan Essences also works with gem elixirs, so the program adds another layer of knowledge and healing. Learn more at www.alaskanessences.com.

Where to Buy Flower Essences

You can find flower essences for purchase in many places. A wonderful variety is available online at various websites, some of which are listed below. Local health food and metaphysical shops may also carry them.

The line of Bach flower remedies is the most common. It includes the Rescue Remedy formula (which includes Impatiens, Star of Bethlehem, Cherry Plum, Rock Rose, and Clematis), which is popular for animals for stress and anxiety relief. You can also take

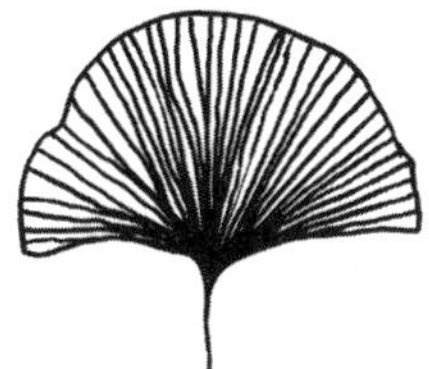

Rescue Remedy as a spray or drops. The Bach remedies also carry a line specifically made for animals, including dogs, cats, horses, and other pets. There is also a Rescue Sleep to aid in sleep disorders and insomnia issues. If you are unsure about which remedies are right for you, many quizzes online can help you discover more about what would work best for you at this time. You can find the Bach remedies at a variety of places online.

The Flower Essence Society (FES), out of Nevada City, California, carries an extensive line of dual-certified organic formulas. They have a variety of individual and combination formulas, including the popular Yarrow Environmental Solution, which helps protect your energetic field from toxins in the environment and is especially helpful for airplane travel. FES has created some specific formulas for caregivers, those in grief, those challenged by fear and anxiety, and so forth. You can find their products and extensive website full of information at www.fesflowers.com.

LotusWei, founded by Katie Hess, has created a line of flower elixirs, anointing oils, serums, bath salts, and more. She has a Feel Good and Transform line of essences, which are infused with honey, so they taste sweet. For example, the Infinite Love formula inspires loving-kindness, magnetism, and self-expression. This formula includes the essence of Hong Kong Orchid, Fireweed, Pink Magnolia, Hawkweed, Lotus, and Pink Tourmaline gem essence. LotusWei also has formulas for quieting the mind, uncovering more joy within, inner peace, radiant energy, inspired action, and much more. Find LotusWei online at www.lotuswei.com.

Desert Alchemy Flower Essences, founded by Cynthia Athina Kemp Scherer in 1983, are crafted from the desert flowers in Arizona, which provides a unique energetic medicine because these plants have had to adapt to an intense environment with periods of little rain. The vibrational imprint of these desert flowers can bring about rapid growth, adaptability, and clarity. Each bottle is made with the intention of utmost care and blessings. Desert Alchemy sells both individual and composite remedies. The composite formulas range from assisting with manifesting abundance to harmonizing addictive patterns. Visit them online at www.desert-alchemy.com.

About the Author

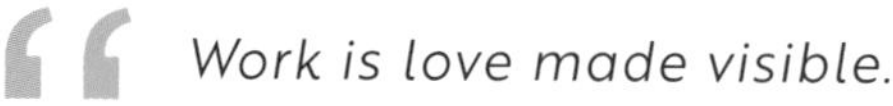

Work is love made visible.

— Khalil Gibran

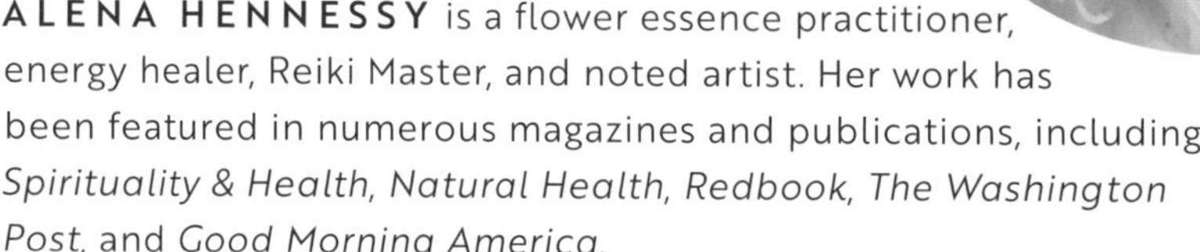

ALENA HENNESSY is a flower essence practitioner, energy healer, Reiki Master, and noted artist. Her work has been featured in numerous magazines and publications, including *Spirituality & Health*, *Natural Health*, *Redbook*, *The Washington Post*, and *Good Morning America*.

She is the author of the Mysteries of Love Oracle Deck, *Cultivating Your Creative Life*, *The Painting Workbook*, and *Intuitive Painting Workshop*. Alena is beloved teacher of the art-making process, both online and at select retreats, and sacred space-holder for women's creative expression. Her paintings combine spiritual inspiration and heartfelt expression with botanical detail. She has exhibited across major cities in the U.S., along with several museum shows.

Acknowledgments

To my family, closest friends, animal companions, and sweet beloved, thank you. I love you dearly and am quite blessed to have you in my life.

I especially want to thank the flowers—for their intricate and countless expressions of beauty. Thank you for all the inspiration, musings, healing, and mystery you provide. This book is of course dedicated to your realm.

About the Artist

JANE HENNESSY credits her formal education as much as the benefit of traveling extensively while with her family for her success. After graduating high school, she received her B.A. from Florida State University, majoring in design and printmaking and art history. Throughout her professional career, she has worked in merchandising design for JC Penny, owned Custom Signs & Murals for twelve years, and later was a digital artist for Fox Television in Tampa, Florida, for nine years.

Jane, mother of three accomplished children, now enjoys painting and living in Asheville, North Carolina. Visit her online at www.janessy.com

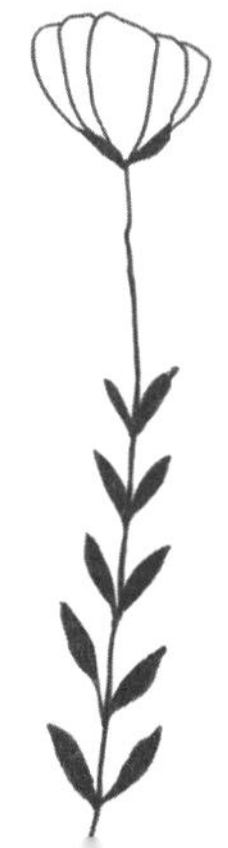

Index

N

O

P

Q

R

S

T

V

W

Y